Anxiety Relief For Kids

On-the-Spot Strategies To Help Your Child Overcome Worry, Panic, And Avoidance

Bridget Flynn Walker, PhD

16pt

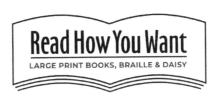

Read How You Want
LARGE PRINT BOOKS, BRAILLE & DAISY

Copyright Page from the Original Book

Publisher's Note

This publication is designed to provide accurate and authoritative information in regard to the subject matter covered. It is sold with the understanding that the publisher is not engaged in rendering psychological, financial, legal, or other professional services. If expert assistance or counseling is needed, the services of a competent professional should be sought.

Distributed in Canada by Raincoast Books

Copyright © 2017 by Bridget Flynn Walker
New Harbinger Publications, Inc.
5674 Shattuck Avenue
Oakland, CA 94609
www.newharbinger.com

Cover design by Amy Shoup

Acquired by Camille Hayes

Edited by Jennifer Eastman

Library of Congress Cataloging-in-Publication Data on file

19   18   17

10   9   8   7   6   5   4   3   2   1   First Printing

TABLE OF CONTENTS

"Bridget Flynn Walker has written a timely book. In our busy pediatric practice, we are seeing an increased number of children with anxiety these days. For parents and professionals alike, she clearly defines the different 'faces' of anxiety, and strategies that can be used to help our children and patients overcome them."
—**Mary D. Piel, MD,** pediatrician at Golden Gate Pediatrics in San Francisco, CA

"This book is a terrific resource for parents of anxious kids! Parents want to know what to do and what not to do to help their child with anxiety. Walker explains how trying to comfort your child can actually be feeding their anxiety. She offers up clear and powerful tools that parents can use with their child that will help them now and for the rest of their lives.
—**Jennifer Shannon, LMFT,** author of *The Anxiety Survival Guide for Teens*

"With warmth and wisdom, this valuable book provides hope and empowerment to parents. Bridget Flynn Walker provides a clear and easily readable understanding of what makes anxiety worse, and scientifically-proven strategies for managing anxiety. Most importantly, she provides a practical road map that parents can follow to help their children become braver and more confident in tackling their fears."

—Aureen Pinto Wagner, PhD, director of The Anxiety Wellness Center in Cary, NC, and author of *Worried No More*

"Just what the doctor ordered! A clear, concise, and practical guide to help parents help their children master their anxieties. I am confronted with patients and their parents every day who are searching for guidance in managing their children's omnipresent worries. The cognitive behavioral therapy (CBT) strategies outlined are easy to understand and straightforward to implement. This book provides a real-life tool kit that will help families and their physicians ease the fears that children often have."

—Laurel J. Schultz, MD, MPH, community pediatrician at Golden Gate Pediatrics, and volunteer associate clinical faculty at the University of California, San Francisco

"Bridget Flynn Walker's book, *Anxiety Relief for Kids,* provides an invaluable resource for parents and mental health professionals to help children manage and overcome anxiety. The book's approach is clear, concise, and informative. This step-by-step guide—full of evidence-based strategies to implement with children—uses easy-to-understand language, and offers vivid examples and helpful worksheets which make the book simple and effective to use."

—Anya Ho, PhD, clinical psychologist at the San Francisco Group for Evidence-Based Psychotherapy

"This book is a much-needed resource for parents of kids with anxiety. It outlines essential psychoeducation about anxiety, and how to tackle its treatment. This book can help empower parents towards addressing their kid's anxiety and give them the essential tools needed to be successful."

—Natalie Todd, PsyD, clinical psychologist at the University of California, San Francisco, working with teens and young adults

"Bridget Flynn Walker's book tackles a complex and vexing problem for so many families, providing simple and easy-to-learn methods that will ease your child's anxiety and boost confidence. *Anxiety Relief for Kids* is a go-to resource for parents or anyone else trying to help a child with excessive anxiety. I recommend it highly."

—Eli Merritt, MD, founder of Merritt Mental Health

"This little gem of a book offers useful information for parents who are first learning about anxiety in their children. The book is highly approachable, and synthesizes much of the currently available information on child anxiety and evidence-based treatment strategies. Parents will particularly appreciate the friendly and unassuming language, and the real-life examples that bring many familiar dilemmas to life. The section on how not to 'feed your child's anxiety' will be especially useful for parents wondering how to help their child feel less anxious without contributing to the kind of unhelpful avoidance that maintains the problem. Bridget Flynn Walker has a clear voice and a knack for explaining ideas so that they just make sense."

—Eli R. Lebowitz, PhD, associate director of the Anxiety and Mood Disorders Program, and assistant professor at the Yale Child Study Center

Foreword

Twenty years ago, my wife and I arrived home from the hospital with our newborn daughter, Madeleine. I turned off the car, and my wife and I sat for a few moments staring in wide-eyed awe at tiny and beautiful Madeleine asleep in her car seat.

I looked at my wife and, with a nervous smile, asked, "By the way, did they give you the operator's manual for the baby?"

My wife looked at me with a nervous—yet less nervous—smile, "No, I thought they gave the manual to you." This did not reassure me.

When I think of that moment, I still think it was a bit crazy, or at least unwise, for the nurse to send us home with a newborn infant. I assume they believed we would figure the parenting thing out, as so many other parents have done, but still, it is unsettling when you think about it, right? Of course, most parents do figure it out, with the support of friends and family members, but what parent has not longed for an operator's manual to guide them at a critical moment in child rearing, particularly at those moments when their child is suffering?

Over 25 percent of children and adolescents suffer with an anxiety disorder, making anxiety disorders the number one mental health issue for youth. Behavioral science tells us that parents play a key role in assisting a child to recover from anxiety disorders and other mental health problems, and it makes intuitive sense too. Parents are in a better position to observe, support, and intervene with their anxious child than any mental health professional. The anxious moments that occur in the lives of most children seldom occur in the therapist's office. They occur in the world in which the child lives—home, school, soccer field, playdates—and, typically, the parents live there too.

So where is the operator's manual for parents who wish to help their child recover from an anxiety disorder? There are many books—or operator's manuals, if you will—on the topic of assisting overanxious children, but perhaps few are as clear and as thoughtful as this one. This book covers the basics of cognitive behavioral therapy (CBT), the psychological treatment of choice for overanxious youth, and the author, Dr. Bridget Flynn Walker, is an expert in this approach.

This book will guide you and your child through the process of recovering from an anxiety disorder. Like any operator's manual, this book covers the basics, such as educating you and your child about anxiety and anxiety disorders, identifying the triggers of your child's anxious response, setting the stage for exposure, and assisting your child in completing and benefiting from these important and essential exposures. Furthermore, although the research on pediatric anxiety disorders and their treatment is extensive and often rather dense for many parents, this book takes some of the most important topics and explains them in simple and straightforward language. Every operator's manual includes a troubleshooting section, and several chapters in this book include one too. In those sections, you will learn strategies to overcome the obstacles that typically arise when helping children face the things that frighten them.

One last point. If, after applying the strategies described in this book, your child continues to suffer, it may be time to find a competent cognitive behavioral therapist who is knowledgeable about pediatric anxiety disorders and knows how to treat them. This book will help with that, too. Having read this book, you will be well prepared to talk with prospective therapists about cognitive behavioral therapy and ask them how they use it to treat their patients. Their answers will tell you who can and cannot help your anxious child. If your child is already meeting with a therapist for help with an anxiety disorder, using this book along with therapy can help your child tremendously. The exercises in this book, particularly the exposure exercises, will greatly supplement therapy sessions, and you and your child can discuss the results of the exercises with your child's therapist. If your child is not engaged in exposure in a systematic manner in therapy, then your child is not receiving CBT, and I would suggest finding another therapist.

Many kids suffer with anxiety disorders, and many kids, through the strategies described in this book, recover from them. Informed, caring, and thoughtful parents play a crucial role in that recovery. Good luck to you as you undertake this important mission to help your child.

—Michael A. Tompkins, PhD
Author, *My Anxious Mind: A Teen's Guide to
Managing Anxiety and Panic*
Codirector, San Francisco Bay Area Center for
Cognitive Therapy
Assistant Clinical Professor of Psychology,
University of California, Berkeley
Oakland, California
November 20, 2016

Introduction

As a parent, you can do a lot to help your anxious child. You can learn how to respond more constructively to your child's distress. You can better understand your child's anxious behaviors so you can make better choices for him. You can even learn how to actively help your child conquer her fears so anxiety no longer creates so much distress and disruption for your child and family. With the program described in this book, you can apply the most up-to-date information scientists have regarding the effective treatment of anxiety problems.

This book presents a program you can use to guide your child toward a happier, healthier life. By providing you with the information and practical tools you need, this easy-to-read primer will show you how to take a more active, constructive, and rewarding role in helping your child manage and, ultimately, overcome anxiety. Whether your child struggles with mild anxious reactions or more difficult anxiety disorders, you have the power to help. As you read this book, you will learn just how critical your role is in this process.

As a clinical psychologist, I have specialized for over fifteen years in using cognitive behavioral therapy (CBT) to successfully and rapidly treat children with anxiety disorders. CBT is a form of psychotherapy that focuses on changing thoughts and behaviors to alleviate emotional problems. Thousands of clinical trials have shown that this approach works, and ongoing research continues to make it even more effective. I have incorporated the latest findings in this book.

CBT is most effective in alleviating the distressing impact of anxiety in children when parents are actively involved in the treatment process (Allen and Rapee 2004; Thirlwall et al. 2013). My own hands-on experience has shown me how pivotal the parents' role is in treating a child's anxiety. In fact, I require parental involvement in each child's treatment because progress tends to be limited when parents are not involved. During the course of treatment, I teach parents about anxiety and how changes to their behavior can help their child.

Getting treatment for your child can be difficult. Many parents have trouble finding a trained clinician in their area, especially one who is taking new patients. The cost of treatment can also be a burden. Fortunately, some studies have suggested that parents can use CBT on their own to help their children. For example, Kerstin Thirlwall and her colleagues in the United Kingdom (2013) found that children whose parents used a self-help book, along with some support from a CBT therapist, were three times more likely to recover than were children who received no treatment.

Although a number of CBT manuals for children with anxiety disorders exist, most are put together in ways that make them difficult for a parent to use successfully. Some present more clinical information than is necessary, making them confusing and overwhelming to a lay person. And none are based in the most current understanding about how to use CBT to treat anxiety problems.

Parents routinely ask me to recommend resources that are evidence based, thorough yet concise, and user friendly that they can use, especially with younger children. I have been hard pressed to identify such a resource. With this in mind, I decided to write *Anxiety Relief for Kids.* In practical, straightforward terms, this book shows you how to share the proven methods of CBT with your child.

This book will not tell you everything there is to know about anxiety disorders in children. That is not my intention, and it isn't necessary for your success. However, it will give you the most crucial information you need to help your child. Specifically, you will learn

- how your child's anxiety starts,
- how your child's anxiety grows,
- what makes your child's anxiety worse,
- what you can do to reduce your child's anxiety,
- how to make better decisions related to your child's anxiety, and
- how to respond more constructively to your anxious child.

I have incorporated the views and experiences of parents into each chapter. The questions a typical parent or child might ask are addressed throughout, and each step is clearly explained so you and your child can feel empowered in the process of successfully managing and conquering anxiety. Easy-to-follow worksheets allow you and your child to work through the program in manageable stages (blank copies of each worksheet are available online). I also include sample conversations that suggest how you might speak with your child at each step.

As you help your child conquer his or her fears, you and your family can expect the quality of your lives to improve. Of course, I can't predict the degree of this change. Some parents will see their child freed from anxiety. Others will make moderate progress, seeing a greater sense of mastery over anxiety symptoms in their child. Yet others will learn from this book about the kind of help their child may need and, with that information, can make sound, educated decisions about which treatment options to pursue for their child. Regardless of which of these best describes your experience, I can promise you will gain knowledge and learn strategies that will move your child closer toward conquering his or her fears.

How to Use This Book

I suggest that you read the chapters of this book in order. I have organized them to help you work through the CBT program in the smoothest and most effective way. This is the order I use when working with patients. The basic knowledge and tools you will need are introduced in the first three chapters. The strategies described in the following chapters build upon one another. If you jump ahead, you may not learn a skill or have some information you need to implement the next step.

Throughout the process, you and your child will be completing a series of worksheets. I have included examples of completed worksheets in the book. Blank worksheets can be downloaded from the publisher's website (http://ww

w.newharbinger.com/39539). You can also find short videos on my website (h ttp://www.drbridgetwalker.com) that illustrate the kinds of conversations you will have with your child.

In my experience, parents who participate actively and complete the worksheets are more successful in helping their child and less likely to engage emotionally in their child's anxiety than are parents who do not. Even if you think you're too busy, I recommend making the time. Devoting just five to ten minutes a day to collecting information about behaviors, for example, will pay dividends in the future, as you and your child learn to deal with anxiety more effectively.

I recommend reading through the book in its entirety before sharing it with your child. You are the leader in this process. If you have a good sense of your goals at each stage and how the work at one stage will help your work at the next, you will be a more effective leader.

The program in this book is designed for children of all ages. I have used it successfully with young children as well as teenagers. That said, you may need to make adaptations depending on the age of your child. For example, you could ask an older child to read the book himself or herself. You will also have to identify the most ageappropriate examples as you develop your own lists of situations, targets, exposures, and rewards.

You know better than anyone else how your child thinks, what he or she likes and dislikes, and how he or she learns. If you keep this in mind as you work through the program, you will have greater success in alleviating the debilitating effects anxiety exerts on your child.

CHAPTER 1

Educate Yourself and Your Child about Anxiety

If you picked up this book, you probably are concerned about your child's well-being and may suspect that anxiety plays a role in your child's suffering. Anxiety can be tough to detect because children who suffer from anxiety problems often do not seem overtly anxious or fearful. Understanding how anxiety appears and how it operates will help you take the first steps toward helping your child.

Anxiety problems can show up in children in a myriad ways. Many parents are baffled by the irrational and exaggerated nature of their child's concerns: Why does Mark habitually believe he's going to bomb his math test in spite of his stellar performances? Why does Tamika insist I reassure her that the doors are locked and the alarm is on even though she knows we live in a safe environment and practice reasonable security precautions every night? How come Francis throws a fit when he can't understand a new concept in science he logically can't be expected to have down yet? Why does Allegra tell me on a daily basis that kids think she's not very smart or funny, when she is one of the more popular children in her class?

Essentially: Why doesn't my child understand reason? Why doesn't she realize that nothing as bad as she predicts ever happens? In other words, why doesn't he learn that his fears are unfounded or greatly exaggerated? I will do my best to answer these questions in this book.

It can be heartbreaking to watch your child struggle with worries that interfere with her activities. Anxiety problems exact tremendous costs on both the sufferer and his or her loved ones—navigating daily life can be exhausting, contentious, and stressful. In this book, I tell you what you need to know about anxiety and how to take concrete steps to help your child conquer his or her anxiety.

The Nature of Anxiety

Many scientists believe anxiety disorders are caused not by the mere presence of fear, but by attempts to escape or control the uncomfortable sensations and thoughts that accompany anxiety—such as a rapid heartbeat or unwanted recurrent thought (Forsyth, Eifert, and Barrios 2006). These tactics are referred to as "avoidance and safety behaviors"—and in the case of obsessive-compulsive disorder, "rituals"—and they typically give anxious individuals short-term relief from anxiety-related distress. The problem is that reliance on these behaviors fuels anxiety over the long term and prevents children from learning that their expectations of dire consequences aren't accurate. This pattern keeps your child trapped in the clutches of anxiety.

Attempts to avoid, suppress, or escape discomfort are often what the parents or teachers of an anxious child notice first. Anxiety can appear as overt worry or fear, accompanied by clear physical signs such as hyperventilation, shaking, and terror. It also often appears as shyness, sensitivity, clinginess, rigidity, quirkiness, oppositionality, low self-confidence, pessimism, indecision, procrastination, and anger. As you can see from table 1, most signs of anxiety are not so obvious. Although the signs may differ, the basic nature of anxiety is the same. Deep down, an anxious child fears being in a particular situation he or she believes will result in a negative consequence. The source of your child's anxiety may not be obvious to you now, but as you read this book, you will learn how to pinpoint what your child fears.

For example, Tom fears going to soccer practice, where he worries an unleashed dog might bite him. His symptoms include a nervous stomach and nausea before practice, and he consistently tells his parents that he just doesn't feel well enough to go. Alicia fears taking tests at school because she worries about getting a less-than-perfect grade. Her symptoms are less obvious than Tom's: she avoids raising her hand in class, in case she gives a wrong answer, and she refuses to participate in any after-school activities that might prevent her from studying.

As a parent, you may observe less obvious signs of avoidance, suppression, and escape behaviors rather than overt anxiety. The important thing to remember is that the underlying nature of anxiety is the same, regardless of how you see it affecting your child, and you will follow the same program to help him or her.

TABLE 1. Signs of Anxiety

Visible Signs of Anxiety	Less Obvious Signs of Anxiety
Physical distress (shaking, crying, hyperventilating, screaming)	Clingy behavior
Fleeing, escaping	Irritability
Outright statements of anxiety ("I'm afraid the house will burn down tonight while I'm asleep.")	Avoidance behavior
	Complaints of physical illness
	Reassurance-seeking behavior
Outright questions expressing fears ("What if you get in a car accident when you go out?")	Argumentative behavior
	Reluctance to try new things (activities, foods, places, routines)
Refusal to engage in activities that cause distress	Extreme shyness, sensitivity
	Being easily distracted
Extreme distress upon contact with feared object (dogs, birds, planes, extreme weather)	Slowness (relative to others of the same age), procrastination
	Overly cautious behavior, indecision
Refusal to be alone or without a parent	Exacting standards
	Sleep difficulties (refusal to sleep alone, go on sleepovers)
	Physical aggression
	Threats of suicide to avoid anxiety-producing situations

Anxiety Disorders Are Common in Children

Anxiety disorders are the most common type of psychological problem children experience; one in eight children suffers from a significant anxiety disorder (Anxiety and Depression Association of America 2016). This means that in an average class of school-aged children, three will suffer from some type of anxiety symptoms that cause significant distress, interfere with their ability to engage in typical activities, or both.

Symptoms can emerge in children as young as four or five, although you may notice symptoms even earlier. Because anxiety can show itself in less-than-obvious ways, many parents are unaware that anxiety is at the root of their child's symptoms or behaviors. As a result, the parents and even a pediatrician or mental health professional may dismiss the symptoms as "developmentally normal" or "just a stage." They may think a child is just shy or overtired or has an attention deficit disorder. Because a young child can't clarify what is happening, and because many mental health professionals are not adequately trained to assess and treat anxiety disorders, it may be years before a correct diagnosis is made and a helpful treatment is found.

Even though parents may not be able to recognize that a child is suffering from anxiety, in my experience, they know their child and know when something feels wrong. My advice is to trust your instincts. If you suspect your child's anxiety adversely affects his or her day-today activities, please use this book as a resource and a guide. I will show you how to take concrete steps to improve your child's life.

The Effects of Anxiety

For starters, is anxiety such a bad thing?

In actuality, some degree of anxiety is a normal part of any healthy person's life. Mother Nature equipped us with the fight-or-flight response to help us protect ourselves in dangerous situations. We have a choice between facing a threat, if we think we can overcome it, or fleeing from it, if we are afraid we can't win. In that case, acting out of fear, in the interest of safety, is a legitimate option. Anxiety can also prove helpful by heightening our performance. All other things being equal, fear of coming in last or losing a game can drive an athlete to perform better than will a less-motivated competitor. Similarly, a student who is a little worried can perform better on a standardized test at school than can a student who couldn't care less about the results.

Often, however, anxiety can grow to the point where, instead of serving us, it becomes harmful to our well-being. This is true of adults as well as children. Not surprisingly, many adults with anxiety problems have endured symptoms since childhood.

Anxiety is considered unhealthy if it keeps a child from living a normal life at home, with friends, and at school. Your child may avoid situations—such as going to public bathrooms, speaking up in class, or being near animals—that spark anxious feelings. Doing this over time tends to increase those fears and eventually impedes healthy psychosocial development and quality of life. Because anxiety symptoms can be masked, children with anxiety disorders often function well in terms of grades, achievement, and more, yet live a tortured internal life rife with worry, fear, or excessive guilt or feelings of responsibility. Over time, high levels of distress and anxiety are mentally and physically exhausting and demoralizing, and a child can become depressed and hopeless about the relentless nature of severe anxiety. In fact, a large body of research tells us that untreated anxiety disorders markedly compromise the quality of life and psychosocial functioning of sufferers (Mendlowicz and Stein 2000; Olatunji, Cisler, and Tolin 2007).

Why It Is Important to Help Your Child Now

Research tells us that if we don't adequately treat children with anxiety disorders, they are more likely to develop other mental illnesses in adulthood, such as depression and substance abuse (Kessler et al. 2005). Furthermore, studies indicate that most anxiety symptoms are chronic; children usually do not simply grow out of them. Unfortunately, the tendency for anxiety to come and go leads parents to believe it will eventually go away once and for all, and so they are disinclined to seek treatment for their child.

Another important reason to help your child conquer anxiety is to prevent it from seemingly becoming integrated into his or her personality. Anxiety is not a personality trait or style, and does not define a person. Personality does not change much over a lifespan, but anxiety symptoms can and do. Not only are anxiety disorders the most common mental health issue, but they are also one of the most treatable. I have seen countless children and adults transformed when their anxiety is treated effectively with CBT.

How Anxiety Operates in Your Child

Before we discuss treatment more, let's look more specifically at how anxiety operates, including the role of family history, the functioning of the brain, and patterns of anxiety.

The Role of Family History

A family history of anxiety issues predisposes a child to such disorders. Although many complex factors, including temperament and environmental influences, are thought to play a role in the development of anxiety disorders, genetic heritability has consistently been found to be a leading risk factor (Beidel and Turner 1997; Kashani et al. 1990; Merikangas, Dierker, and Szatmari 1998). In fact, Dr. Armen Goenjian and his colleagues at UCLA (2014) pinpointed two genes that increase the risk for posttraumatic stress disorder (PTSD). Not everyone who has those genes will get PTSD, but having them increases the odds. Similar findings may someday be revealed for other anxiety disorders.

Rarely do I treat a child for anxiety who does not have relatives with a history of anxiety. Many parents readily report they suffer from it, while others are unaware it runs in their family, because the sufferers arranged their lives to avoid situations that triggered their fears, or they engaged in behaviors that mitigated their exposure to such situations. Such relatives may simply be considered eccentric or control freaks. Just as you know your child may inherit your predisposition to allergies, it can be helpful to know that he or she may share your or your family's vulnerability to anxiety.

EXERCISE: Identifying Genetic History. If you haven't done so already, I suggest you take some time to consider whether anyone who is genetically related to your child suffers from anxiety. Talk to members of your family—your siblings and parents and others. Be sure to do this without introducing either blame or shame; your purpose is simply to gather information and gain clarity so you can help your child.

Although we do not fully understand the complex hereditary and environmental factors that contribute to the development of anxiety disorders, scientific research is making the picture more clear. In fact, leading researchers have developed programs to help prevent those at risk due to genetic factors from developing anxiety disorders (Ginsberg 2009).

I do not mean to suggest that genes or family history are the only factors in the development of an anxiety disorder, but it is an important thing to consider. Your child's anxiety is probably not caused by bad parenting or traumatic events, especially if your child has not been neglected, traumatized, or abused. I stress this because many therapists have traditionally looked for trauma as the cause of anxiety in both children and adults. The empirical data simply do not support this point of view.

Anxiety Comes in Spikes

Hundreds of neuroimaging studies have been conducted over the past fifteen years comparing the brain anatomy and functioning of individuals suffering from anxiety disorders with those of non-sufferers. This research confirms the involvement of distinct parts of the brain, including the basal ganglia, amygdala, and hippocampus (Holzschneider and Mulert 2011). Of course, current technology does not allow us to use brain scans to diagnose the disorder. But we do know from these studies and from the clinical and subjective reports of sufferers that anxiety comes in *spikes.* These spikes represent the increased and prolonged activity of the brain structures, such as the amygdala, responsible for the fear and anxiety response that results when a child is exposed to a trigger. As long as the amygdala is activated, the child experiences fear and anxiety. When the amygdala calms down, the distressing emotions pass. This helps us to understand how a child experiences anxiety and explains the curious nature of anxiety.

Children who suffer from anxiety usually realize intellectually that their fears are extreme or even completely irrational. We call this *insight.* However, when a child is in the midst of a spike, this insight erodes, and he believes his fears are real and justified for the duration of that spike. After the spike has passed, he tends to regain insight. Consider this example.

Joseph is a twelve-year-old who attends a top-notch private boys' school.

He gets straight As, plays a team sport each season, and participates in a demanding choir program. His parents worry that he takes life too seriously and doesn't have much fun. When they encourage him to just hang out with his friends, he reassures them he is fine with the way things are and has no time to do things that are not constructive.

Frequently, Joe becomes worried he will not have time for everything he has to do. During these periods, his parents brace for heartbreaking crying fits as Joe sobs that he will be unable to memorize his music or complete a big homework assignment. His parents remind him that he often has these fears and always manages to get his work done, and even to get perfect grades and good feedback from his choirmaster.

In these moments of anxiety, Joe does not—and, in fact, cannot—see the evidence of past successes his parents present to him. He cries, "This is different, Mom!" Even when his parents remind him that he frequently tells them each particular situation is uniquely dire and yet it still works out just fine, he can't make use of this logic in the moment.

After Joe has performed his songs in the choir and turned in his assignments, his anxiety passes. He tells his parents they were right and acknowledges that he need not worry as much as he does. In fact, he vows he will handle the next situation differently. Although Joe and his parents hope he will learn from this experience, unfortunately, his anxiety resurfaces the next time he faces this type of situation.

Anxiety Tends to Wax and Wane

Anxiety symptoms tend to fluctuate across time and situations. Whereas spikes refer to the fluctuation in anxiety during a period in which one is experiencing symptoms, the waxing and waning of anxiety can span a lifetime. Over some weeks or months, your child may experience fewer or less intense worries than over other weeks or months. Some situations will trigger your child's fears, while others will not. For example, Joseph, with his perfectionist worries about academic performance, may study excessively during the school year, checking and rechecking assignments, having meltdowns, seeking reassurance from parents or teachers about the quality of his work, and worrying about getting enough sleep to keep up his performance. Once summer arrives, these worries may disappear, only to return when summer comes to an end and any summer homework is due.

Anxious Children Tend to Interpret Even Safe Situations As Dangerous

Children who are predisposed to anxiety tend to notice potential threats in situations other children would not consider threatening (Craske et al. 2008; Lissek et al. 2010). For example, an anxious child might panic when a fire truck drives by, while another child might look at that truck with excitement. Because anxious children interpret more situations as threatening, they tend to be on high alert for potential danger in their daily lives. The more they look for potential danger, the more they notice threats and the more anxious they feel.

We know from numerous studies that this cognitive bias increases the likelihood of anxiety problems developing, and it exacerbates anxiety problems once they have started. Furthermore, it interferes with a child's ability to learn that particular situations need not be feared.

Anxious Children Don't Usually Learn from Experience

Think about how you have learned from mistakes that had consequences. I, for one, have never forgotten what earned me my first traffic violation and the financial impact of being late on a credit card payment. At all ages, we learn from our experiences. However, children who are predisposed to anxiety do not learn in this way from their experiences. They have a deficit that interferes with what learning theorists call "inhibitory learning" (Craske et al. 2015). This means that, despite numerous experiences in feared situations in which no negative consequences occur, these children don't learn to be less afraid. Their new learning does not correct their prior learning.

For example, each and every time Joseph's brain calms down after an anxiety spike, he has a rational understanding that his fears were not well founded. He totally gets it, but he still can't learn from all of his successes. The most current research tells us that for CBT to be effective with Joe and other anxious children, we must also address their inability to learn from the experience.

"My Child's Worries Are Like a Game of Whack-A-Mole."

It is common for an anxious child to be focused on a particular worry only to have another fear pop up and trump that worry. When a child's worries shift from one thing to another, parents are often exasperated and confused. It doesn't make logical sense. It's like a game of Whack-A-Mole, and they are frustrated at the impossible task of conquering all the individual sources of anxiety for their child.

Not all children with anxiety experience equally frequent shifts in focus, but it is normal for anxiety to operate in this way. Understanding this general tendency will help you help your child better. If your child's worries shift focus frequently, make an effort to take that in stride. Though this might feel frustrating and overwhelming, try to accept this as part of your child's unique presentation.

SUMMARY: What Did You Learn from This Chapter?

At the end of every chapter, I summarize the highlights of what we have covered. I suggest you discuss with your child's other parent—or write down for yourself—what you learned from the chapter and how it applies to your child. Taking a moment to do this will help your rain consolidate new learning, so you will be more likely to have access to it when you need it. This will also set the tone for the work you do with your child in conquering his or her anxiety. You will be asking your son or daughter, "What did you learn?" frequently in this program. Here is some of what I hope you learned from this chapter:

- Anxiety can show itself in a myriad ways in children—irritability, clinginess, aggression, avoidance, indecision, and procrastination—that don't necessarily scream *anxiety.*
- Anxiety problems are very common in children and are, in fact, the most common psychological problem children experience.
- Untreated anxiety often has serious and negative impacts on children's well-being, quality of life, and development. Ultimately, they can increase the likelihood of more serious mental disorders in adulthood.
- Evidence suggests the genetic transmission of predispositions for anxiety. It runs in families.

- Anxiety comes in spikes that are usually triggered by particular situations.
- Most children have insight about their anxiety. They have the capacity to see that their fears are either completely irrational or at least greatly exaggerated.
- Over time—even over a lifetime—anxiety symptoms wax and wane.
- Anxious children are born with neurobiological tendencies that lead them to perceive danger even in neutral situations.
- Anxious children have learning deficits that make it difficult for them to learn to be less fearful after a feared consequence did not occur.
- Some children have worries that fluctuate a great deal. This is normal.

CHAPTER 2

Determine If Your Child Has an Anxiety Problem

Because anxiety symptoms often are not obvious, it can be challenging to know if anxiety is the true root of your child's problem. The questionnaire in the first section of this chapter is designed to help you gain this level of clarity. The next step is becoming familiar with what you can do to intervene. The remaining sections of this chapter present an overview of the CBT approach and how you can implement it in your child's life.

Is My Child's Anxiety Unhealthy?

Your intuition as a parent has probably already helped you get a sense of your child's level of anxiety. While this intuition is very valuable, it's not usually enough to determine if a child's behavior indicates an unhealthy degree of anxiety.

EXERCISE: Assessing Your Child's Anxiety. The following questionnaire lists behaviors commonly observed by parents of anxious children. Read each question and answer yes or no, based on your observations of your child.

Does your child...

- repeatedly ask "what if" questions and, despite constant reassurance, continue to worry?
- refuse to sleep in his own room, becoming distressed and agitated when asked to do so?
- avoid particular situations, such as movie theaters, restaurants, crowded places, noisy environments, or parks?
- refuse to eat many foods, limiting herself to foods she feels comfortable with?
- engage in behaviors repeatedly to quell his distress?

- require you to say certain statements in particular ways or do some things in specific manners?
- worry about making errors or missing assignments to the point of frequently reviewing work, seeking reassurance from you that the work is satisfactory, or repeatedly checking her backpack or daily planner?
- procrastinate excessively on schoolwork or other obligations in spite of the fact that he demonstrates competence in completing them?
- experience great difficulty making decisions and worry about whether a decision is the "best" or "right" one?
- fear anything less than a perfect performance in academic or athletic situations?
- refuse to discard unnecessary items due to fears of needing items in the future or because they have sentimental value?
- become distressed when separated from you, refusing to be left with

a babysitter or to go on sleepovers or overnight trips without you?

- express fear of germs, diseases, or dirt to the point of avoiding public restrooms, shopping carts, or doorknobs and washing her hands or using hand sanitizers excessively?
- refuse to go to school?
- refuse to raise his hand in class or speak in front of classmates?
- exhibit extreme shyness that inhibits social interactions?
- exhibit distressing physiological manifestations of anxiety, such as shaking, hyperventilating, becoming nauseated, or feeling lightheaded?
- express excessive or inappropriate guilt or sense of responsibility?

If you answered yes to one or more of these questions, it is likely your child is manifesting anxiety that is severe enough to warrant intervention. Keep in mind that this list may not capture your child's unique presentation. Your child may exhibit behaviors similar to those listed here without matching them exactly.

Please note that answering yes to several questions in the exercise is not a formal diagnosis. You should not try to diagnose an anxiety disorder based on this simple questionnaire. Rather, I intend it as a tool to suggest possible next steps. Keep in mind that, as we discussed in the previous chapter, some degree of anxiety is normal for everyone. Your focus here should be on determining whether your child engages in these behaviors enough to be deemed a problem. Do the behaviors you have observed cause your child a significant level of distress? Do they interfere with your child's comfortable participation in normal activities?

If you answer these secondary questions in the affirmative, it is time to take action. If you have concerns, it is not premature to intervene. Getting help can only benefit your child; there is zero risk in addressing these issues now. In fact, all the recommendations in this book are intended to make your child a stronger, more mentally flexible, and resilient person.

Cognitive Behavioral Therapy

Let's assume you believe—from what you have learned thus far about anxiety and from answering the brief questionnaire—that your child is exhibiting symptoms of unhealthy anxiety. Your first response is likely to take him to his pediatrician or to a child therapist for a professional evaluation. This is a reasonable step to take. Unfortunately—and surprisingly—you may find that you do not get the help you need. For example, your pediatrician may simply advise you to wait for him to "grow out of it." Or play therapy may be recommended to "get to the root of the problem causing the anxiety." Neither of these courses of action is based on any solid evidence of efficacy. A psychiatrist might prescribe medication as the first course of action, even though it is not recommended by the National Institute of Mental Health or by most providers with expertise in treating anxiety orders. Unfortunately, many mental health professionals are not adequately trained to assess and treat anxiety disorders effectively.

The course of action recommended by most mental health professionals and endorsed by the National Institute of Mental Health and other scholarly organizations, such as the Anxiety and Depression Association of America and the International OCD Foundation, is cognitive behavioral therapy (CBT). In some cases, medication is prescribed in addition. More than 70 percent of the children I treat respond well to CBT alone and do not need medication. I suggest you use the knowledge you are gaining from this book to help guide you to get the most effective help.

Overview of the CBT Approach

CBT originated in the 1970s through the integration of behavior therapy and cognitive therapy. Behavior therapy, developed by B.F. Skinner, PhD, in the 1950s, focuses on how concrete behaviors either reinforce or extinguish negative emotional states. It explains how we learn complex emotional and behavioral patterns and how we can relearn them. Cognitive therapy, developed by Aaron Beck, MD, in the 1960s, centers on thought patterns and is concerned with identifying and modifying dysfunctional or irrational thinking that can exacerbate and maintain negative emotional states.

The basic tenet of CBT is that if we can learn to change our dysfunctional thinking and the behaviors that reinforce negative emotional states, we will feel better. This involves identifying distorted thinking, changing those thoughts, and adjusting specific behaviors.

CBT is the most highly researched form of psychotherapy. Indeed, one of the greatest strengths of CBT is that it is based on so much evidence. Thousands of carefully controlled studies support its efficacy. All this research means CBT has evolved in ways that allow us to help patients more effectively now than we could even a few years ago. This is especially true with respect to the use of CBT in treating anxiety disorders.

Before I explain the specific process of using CBT, it is critical to understand some of the basic scientific principles behind it. Without this information, the treatment can appear at first glance to be counterintuitive, especially with respect to anxiety disorders. In fact, the actions you and your child are currently taking in response to anxiety may be the opposite of what I am going to propose you do. Sometimes trusting your instincts can lead you to unintentionally exacerbate the problem. If this sounds confusing, my advice is to trust the science.

Exposures

Gradual, repeated *exposure* to the situations that trigger your child's fears is the central component of effective CBT for anxiety disorders. The main goal of exposures is to learn something new. Your child learns to overcome the deficit I discussed in chapter 1 that hinders him from learning that his fears are not realistic. By repeatedly confronting the fearful situation, he discovers that the frightening consequences that were anticipated do not actually come to fruition—or that if consequences do occur, they are not as bad as were expected. This type of learning is facilitated by the arousal that occurs when confronting the fear. Conversely, it won't occur when a child avoids the situations that trigger anxiety.

When I explain the exposure model to parents, they often say something like this: "But Sarah is exposed to that situation all the time. Nothing changes! She still complains and is worried about raising her hand in class. She just won't do it! How can the exposures you're talking about really work?" Take a deep breath and read on.

The science behind the therapeutic use of exposure is impressive (Abramowitz 2013). Studies consistently show that parts of the brain, such as the amygdala, that are overactive in people with anxiety problems become significantly less active after exposure therapy. Clinically, this correlates with a significant reduction in anxiety symptoms. As our knowledge of the brain continues to grow, evidence of the efficacy of exposure therapies mounts. For example, researchers at the Reijmers Lab at Tufts University found that exposure therapy silenced the so-called fear neurons in the brains of mice who were put into fearful situations (Trouche et al. 2013). In fact, exposure therapy actually remodeled the brain—the brain did not just *react* differently during exposure therapy, but it was *rewired* to react differently in future situations. Although this particular study has not been done in humans, research like this is helping us understand what makes exposure therapy effective for so many people.

How we do exposure therapy has been evolving, based on the latest research. For the past three decades, psychologists operated under the assumption that exposure therapy works by replacing fear-based learning with new learning through the process of *habituation* (Rachman 1980). Habituation means becoming accustomed to something; in exposure therapy, it means having less of a reaction to whatever triggers anxiety, and thus lowering fear. For example, if a child fears off-leash dogs, I might start with an exposure in which she views a video of off-leash dogs multiple times. Fear-based learning will cause her to have a strong fear response to the first viewing. But with repeated viewings, this fear response will reduce. At this point, we would say she has habituated to the video of off-leash dogs. The old model understood this to mean that new learning had replaced the old fear-based learning.

More recently, this model was updated by researchers who noticed that, while habituation does reliably occur with exposure therapy, some individuals relapse. This led them to question, why would relapse occur if old fear-based learning has been replaced by new learning? Michelle Craske and others (2015) studied this and demonstrated that although it may be preempted by new learning, the old learning does not disappear. It can resurface in another anxiety-provoking situation. Therefore, treatment can't simply rely on habituation.

Another problem with the old model is its focus on fear reduction. Saying the goal of exposures is to *eliminate* fear sends the message that anxiety is bad and can't be tolerated. This is neither true nor realistic. A child who learns to tolerate some degree of anxiety is less likely to fear it and therefore less likely to experience spikes in anxiety than is one who is trying unsuccessfully to eliminate all anxiety.

In chapters 8 and 9, you will learn to guide your child through exposures, and you will be shown how to maximize the likelihood that new learning will inhibit the old learning.

Education to Manage Anxiety for a Lifetime

Not only will the strategies in this book help your child manage troubling anxiety symptoms, but you and your child will also acquire skills, knowledge, and tools to be used for a lifetime. In this chapter, we have begun the process by examining some of the basic science behind CBT and exposure therapy. This is an education both for you as a parent and for your child. Both of you need to have a clear understanding about what you are embarking on for this program to be most effective. This means understanding what exposures are, how they work, and how you will be helping your child implement them. This knowledge will give you the confidence you need to follow and adhere to the strategies outlined in the chapters that follow.

SUMMARY: What Did You Learn from This Chapter?

- You can observe your child's behavior to determine whether he has an unhealthy level of anxiety. These behaviors include not being reassured by answers to "what if" questions, not sleeping in his own room, worrying excessively about homework, and procrastinating.
- If a child's anxiety interferes with her ability to engage in typical age-appropriate activities or causes a great deal of distress, she probably has a problem severe enough to warrant treatment.
- CBT is the gold standard for effective treatment of anxiety problems in children. Its method

has evolved over the past decade, resulting in improved efficacy.

- CBT is evidence based and is the most highly researched type of therapy.
- Gradual, repeated, and varied exposures to the situations that trigger a child's fears form the central component of effective CBT for anxiety.
- "Habituation" refers to a reduction of the fear response during exposure. Recent research questions the value of fear reduction as the primary goal of exposure therapy and suggest that children should also learn to tolerate some degree of fear.

CHAPTER 3

Create a Toolbox

As with any endeavor, the proper tools can make a project easier. As a first step in the program outlined in this book, I am going to introduce you to the basic tools you and your child will be using throughout. These include the fear thermometer, worry hill, the candy jar, nickname the fear, rewards, and smart talk. As you will see, putting some of these tools to use requires multiple steps. Thus, you will actually be embarking on the program as you work through this chapter.

Fear Thermometer

The fear thermometer allows both parent and child to assess the level of fear or distress the child feels in a given situation. This tool has been widely used in treating anxiety for many years (March and Mulle 1998). In my experience, children of all ages readily grasp the concept of the fear thermometer and use it easily. You and your child will use the fear thermometer to

- collect data about the level of fear or distress she experiences,
- gain objectivity about her anxious feelings,
- communicate with each other without becoming overly emotional, and
- plan exposures.

As figure 1 shows, a 10 on the fear thermometer indicates the greatest level of distress and a 1 the lowest. The goal is for your child to assess his degree of fear when experiencing an anxious reaction. Your child will provide a subjective rating of the degree of fear, distress, or discomfort he is experiencing in that particular situation. Alternatively, you can estimate the level of fear he experiences in that situation. Children typically say a fear rating of 10 corresponds with such anxiety that they will avoid the situation altogether or tolerate it with extreme distress.

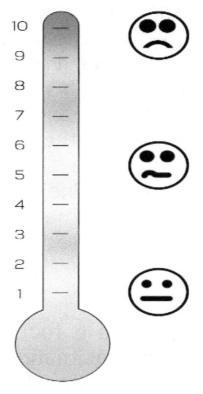

Figure 1. The Fear Thermometer

There are no right or wrong fear thermometer readings, but you want to understand your child's perceptions as accurately as possible. In other words, find out what constitutes a 10 for him, what constitutes a 9, 8, 7, and so on. As you begin to use the fear thermometer with your child, ask enough questions so you can both feel you are on the same page.

I encourage you and your child to make friends with the fear thermometer because you will use it extensively as he learns to conquer his fears. Keep it simple and convey a matter-of-fact attitude about using the thermometer. The more you use it, the more comfortable and routine it will feel. I love the fear thermometer because it is so very simple, versatile, and useful.

Worry Hill

The worry hill is a tool to illustrate to your child how habituation works and to motivate participation in exposures. I borrowed the term "worry hill" from Aureen Pinto Wagner (2005), who used it to make the concepts of exposure and CBT more accessible to children. The worry hill is used in conjunction with the fear thermometer. The vertical axis presents fear thermometer ratings, that is, the level of anxiety or distress in a given situation. The horizontal axis represents the number or exposures or the duration of a single exposure (figure 2).

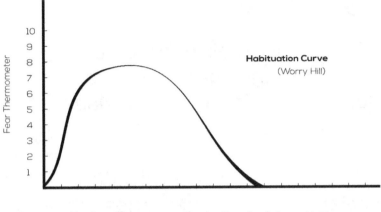

Figure 2. The Worry Hill (the Habituation Curve). Reprinted with permission from Aureen Pinto Wagner, PhD. Worry Hill® is registered in the U.S. Trademark and Patent Office.

Even children who are too young to understand math can grasp what it means to go up and down the worry hill. Use the graphic to show your child how she climbs up the left side of the worry hill when anxiety rises in a fearful situation. You can walk your fingers up the hill to show how her anxiety reaches a peak and then down the other side as anxiety declines and habituation occurs. This helps your child understand that anxiety may get worse when doing beginning exposures, but it will get better in the long term.

The Candy Jar

I use the metaphor of a candy jar to explain the goal of exposures to children; it helps children visualize and understand the usefulness of forming new memories. The candy jar is your child's brain, filled with his various associations and memories related to feared situations.

Each green candy represents one that is nonthreatening, and each red candy represents one that feels threating or dangerous. For example, if your child fears dogs, we would expect him to have more red than green candies related to dogs. The red candies might stand for his many associations (not necessarily based on real experience) with dogs that bite, snarl, or bark loudly, while a green candy might stand for a cute sleeping puppy. In this case, the goal of exposures would be to form new nonthreatening associations and memories about being near dogs. Each worry hill your child climbs related to dogs will add a green candy to his brain. The more green candies your child has, the more likely he will pull a green one from his brain when he encounters a dog, and hence feel at ease rather than terrified.

I recommend introducing the worry hill and the candy jar together. Think of it this way: your child will need to climb lots of worry hills to add enough green candies to the candy jar so he will be likely to pull a green candy rather than a red candy in previously feared situations. The red candies will still be there, but the goal is to overpower the red ones with green ones.

Nickname the Fear

Nicknaming can help both you and your child maintain objectivity and get a handle on her fears. A nickname provides a constructive way to refer to anxiety, rather than engaging in behaviors that feed her fears. Recall from chapter 1 that anxiety tends to come in spikes and your child is more likely to believe her fears during a spike than after that spike passes. Using a nickname to refer to a fear puts you and your child in a position of control because it reminds both of you that her brain is in a spike.

Nicknaming a fear also fosters a neutral attitude about anxiety. No one likes having strong feelings of anxiety, and children can naturally develop a negative attitude toward their anxiety. This attitude only intensifies the anxiety—research shows that when children are less negative about a particular fear, they experience less distress and are able to make greater gains from exposure therapy (Zbozinek, Holmes, and Craske 2015).

Start Using the Tool of Nicknaming

To use this tool, ask your child to come up with a nickname for her fears and anxiety, one that is simple and direct. It should have meaning to your child, and it should be lighthearted and not frightening or negative. For example, a child who fears germs might select Germ Worm or Germster. You and your child will use this nickname as much as possible when anxiety is triggered.

After your child decides on a nickname, help her learn to use it. When she has a high fear thermometer rating, she should think to herself, *Hi, Germ Worm!* Using the nickname should be done mostly silently because children sometimes create a ritual around the nickname when they repeatedly speak it aloud. This practice can interfere with recovery and will be discussed in chapter 5.

The goal is simply to have your child tag and greet the fear each time in an objective manner. You don't want her to think things such as *Go away, Germ Worm!* or *I hate you, Germ Worm!* or *You suck, Germ Worm!* The idea is to remain objective, without adding more negative thoughts. The more readily your child can respond to anxiety by identifying it with a nickname, the more easily she can view the bad feelings in a healthier way. Some children find that nicknaming alone helps them a great deal.

You can introduce the nickname tool to your child with the following exercise, which involves imagination.

EXERCISE: Trying Out a Nickname. If your child is fearful of germs, for example, suggest imagining being in a situation in which it is necessary to touch a doorknob she believes is not clean. Ask if she feels her fear thermometer rating rise when picturing herself touching the knob. Just imagining being in the situation may be enough for this to happen. If so, that's great. When your child feels anxiety developing, instruct her to say silently, *Hi, Germ Worm.* Tell her to use the nickname whenever her fear thermometer rating rises in real life.

How You As a Parent Can Help

You should regularly encourage and reward the use of nicknaming. (Rewards are discussed later in this chapter.) Set up a time each day when you can talk to your child about the nicknaming. Is your child nicknaming 50 percent of the time when the fear is triggered? More frequently or less frequently? The goal is for your child to consistently use the nickname whenever anxiety is triggered. Don't punish or castigate your child for not meeting the hoped-for frequency of usage. You do not want to express any disappointment; instead, show support for successful nicknaming even if progress is slow at first.

You should use the nickname when speaking to your child about a fear response. If you see her beginning to exhibit an anxious response, assist by asking, in a calm and businesslike voice, "Is that Germ Worm?" This prodding can be a useful reminder to her—not only are you reinforcing the nicknaming, but you are also modeling an objective, composed, and accepting response to anxiety.

Don't be surprised if your child occasionally rebuffs your attempts to use the nickname. I hear from many parents and children alike that the child sometimes can't maintain insight during a spike. The child may respond with frustration: "No, it's not Worry Bug!" In times like these, remember that less is more. Refrain from trying to convince him it is indeed Worry Bug. Wait a bit to respond, and allow him the chance to sort it out. By doing so, you are less likely to engage in behaviors that unintentionally feed his fears. You also model a neutral, calm, and constructive attitude about anxiety.

Because nicknaming a worry asks your child to move closer (i.e., be exposed) to that fear, he may worry that this will lead to more thoughts about worries in general, and thus create more anxiety. Initially, this may occur. He may have more thoughts about worries in the short run. And as he begins to face his fears, feelings of distress will arise. But over the long run, the more your child faces his fears, the less anxious he will be.

Some parents question whether an older child will find nicknaming silly or infantile. In my experience, a motivated teenager will not object to nicknaming, primarily because he can choose the name himself and because it is a tool that is employed in silence. Whatever name the teen has chosen is usually not shared with anyone other than the parents, and therefore it is easy to implement the tool in a private manner.

The Nickname Game

Here's a game you can play with your child at any age to help him practice nicknaming. There are two roles: the worry and the nickname. Take turns playing these two roles.

Whoever plays the role of the worry speaks first. That person must verbalize what the worry says to the child that makes him scared. For example, if I play the role of the worry, I might say, "John, if you touch that shopping cart, you'll get germs on you."

John, in the nickname role, says aloud, "Hi, Germ Worm."

I might continue with, "If you can't wash your hands right away with special soap, you'll feel super worried and won't be able to focus with your tutor."

John would reply, "Hi, Germ Worm."

After a few repetitions, switch roles. Try to have fun with this game. See who is fastest at interrupting Germ Worm with the nickname.

I play this game with my patients to make sure they understand how to use the nickname. It is a good way to break the ice, so they are prepared and not worried about using the nickname.

Rewards

You should create incentives that will encourage your child to use her CBT toolbox. Children vary: some feel motivated to make these changes and require little incentive; others need more inducement. You need to gauge the level of your child's motivation. Even with a highly motivated child, I recommend establishing a reward system. I discuss the use of rewards in detail in chapter 6; for now, here are a few general guidelines.

It is crucial that the prize be delivered in a timely fashion; therefore, you must select a reward you are certain you can provide—and promptly. For example, if you promise a trip to visit the cousins but know it will be difficult to get away, choose a different incentive.

Additionally, when selecting a reward, focus on your child's desires. You may ask her for a list of proposed incentives, but ultimately you must make the decision about what is an appropriate reward. Remember, a child must desire the reward enough that she is willing to do the challenging work.

Be careful when using point systems. Preteens and teens have the cognitive ability to appreciate delayed gratification. Depending on their maturity level, they may be willing to accumulate symbolic rewards while waiting for a bigger pay-off. However, a point system does not work effectively for children in the five-to ten-year range. I suggest parents decide on a physical reward that can be delivered immediately when dealing with this younger age group. An ice cream cone, twenty minutes of online time, a trip to the park, and a small toy are examples of immediate rewards.

You need to acknowledge that this is hard work for your child. The reward system must be planned in advance. You do not want to treat it as an afterthought or a last-ditch effort to encourage cooperation. If your child resists, and then you propose a reward system after your initial monitoring has failed, the reward can feel like bribery.

Instead, treat the reward in a matter-of-fact way. Be careful not to over-reward at this point, because a reluctant child will need even larger rewards as treatment becomes more difficult.

Smart Talk

A powerful tool in your CBT toolbox is what I call *smart talk.* It is one way to help your child learn to correct the kind of irrational thinking that accompanies fear and anxiety. Because smart talk is more complex than the other tools covered in this chapter, I devote chapter 7 to it. Even though smart talk may initially seem harder to learn than some of the more basic tools, after your child becomes familiar with it, she will be able to call upon it as readily and automatically as any of the other tools.

SUMMARY: What Did You Learn from This Chapter?

- The main tools in your child's toolbox include the fear

thermometer, worry hill, candy jar, nicknaming, rewards, and smart talk.

- The fear thermometer allows you and your child to assess the level of fear or distress your child feels in a given situation.
- The worry hill and candy jar help your child understand how and why exposures work.
- A nickname is a label that provides a constructive way to refer to anxiety.
- Nicknaming can help both you and your child maintain objectivity and get a handle on his fears.
- You should use rewards to incentivize your child to use her CBT toolbox.
- Smart talk is a tool your child can use to correct the kind of irrational thinking that accompanies fear and anxiety.

CHAPTER 4

Identify Triggers and Determine the Fear

In this chapter, you will begin to put the tools in your toolbox to use as you become acquainted with the main processes you and your child will use in this program. In particular, I will describe trigger situations, monitoring, and the downward arrow technique. These are essential elements in planning exposures for your child.

Trigger Situations

When your child responds with anxiety in specific situations, it means he or she fears particular consequences of being in those situations. Some children suffer from acute episodes of anxiety that seem to come out of the blue and are accompanied by strong physical symptoms (a racing heart, trembling, dizziness, choking sensations, chest tightness, and nausea). You will learn how to address these kinds of panic attacks in chapter 8. Most children, however, do not experience anxiety as a free-floating feeling that attacks without reason. Even if they are not certain exactly what it is, something triggers their anxious response. It could be waiting for the bus in the morning. It could be discarding a simple and useless item. It could be sleeping alone in a room. It could be raising a hand in class. It could be receiving a quiz or test back from the teacher and seeing what the grade is. So the first step in addressing anxiety is to identify the specific triggers.

Many parents who bring a child in for treatment are readily able to identify the situations that trigger their child's anxiety. Other parents have a harder time and need more guidance. I find that when parents learn more about how anxiety behaves, they become better at identifying these triggers and the many subtle variations in a situation that trigger different levels of fear.

Once triggers have been identified, the specific content or structure of the fear must be clarified. What does your child think will happen when he is in a trigger situation? Identifying the content or structure is not usually as obvious to parents as are the triggers. For example, parents may be aware that their child becomes worried when he is called upon to answer a question in class. He may try to avoid being called on by slouching in his chair, looking down, and allowing his hair to partially hide his face. In this case, the trigger is clear—being called upon—but the parents don't know specifically what about it frightens him.

Even when they ask him, "Why does talking in front of the class worry you?" they are likely to get a vague answer: "I just don't like talking in front of everybody." Parents often leave it at that and simply assume their child is shy. The content of the fear remains a mystery, but identifying the content is vital for helping your child. For example, he may have fears of being judged negatively by others (social anxiety) or may have perfectionist worries and feel terrified about giving a wrong answer.

This chapter shows you step-by-step how to identify the situations that trigger your child's anxiety and how to determine what she fears about being in these situations. Identifying both the triggers and the content of your child's fears is vital in the process of helping your child conquer her fears. There is a great deal to know about the specifics of your child's fears, so this is not a process you should try to rush through.

The best way to determine the triggers is to observe your child and determine the situations in which she becomes distressed, worried, or avoidant. For starters, ask yourself the following questions:

- In which situations does my child become distressed?
- Does my child avoid any situations?
- Is my child distressed in situations that previously were not problematic?

If this points you straight to all your child's triggers—great. However, remember that your child may not have obvious signs of anxiety (see table 1 in chapter 1). For example, she may attempt to convince you she simply no longer likes playing soccer, rather than admit to being terrified of being bitten by an off-leash dog in the park where practice is held. Or she might start to avoid certain social situations by making excuses you find illogical or strange. Because a good proportion of children do not show obvious signs of anxiety, a little more detective work on your part may be necessary. This starts with monitoring.

Monitoring

Monitoring involves both observing the situations in which your child experiences anxiety and noting how you respond in these situations. The purpose is to accumulate data about both your child's and your behaviors. Monitoring also begins to put some parameters around your child's anxious behaviors, which shifts his focus from fearing anxiety—and whatever situation triggers it—to learning to manage and conquer it.

The information gathered using a Parent Monitoring Worksheet includes the date, the situation, the behavior observed, your response, and your child's level of distress (as estimated by you) gauged on a scale from 1 to 10. You will use this information later to help you change any of your behaviors that may be contributing to your child's anxiety. Here is an example of the information eleven-year-old Sally's parent noted on her Parent Monitoring Worksheet.

February 11

Situation: *Sally was working on an oral report and started to cry about going to school tomorrow.*

What I observed about my child: *She said she didn't think she could do her report because "it's so bad, everyone will think I'm stupid if I do it." She sobbed and begged me to let her stay home or get her teacher to allow her to do it in writing instead.*

How I responded: *I asked her to practice in front of me after she calmed down a little. She did fine, but when I said I thought she was ready to give the report in class, she became upset again. I tried to explain that no one does a perfect job, and*

some will be better than others. That did not comfort her at all.
Fear thermometer number: *9*

February 12
Situation: *Eating breakfast and getting ready for school.*
What I observed about my child: *She said she felt really sick and thought she was going to throw up. She said she thought she had a fever and needed to stay home from school.*
How I responded: *I talked to Sally about how everyone has nerves about presenting to a group. I took her temperature, and she didn't have a fever. She denied feeling sick because of anxiety. I made her go to school.*
Fear thermometer number: *8*

February 12
Situation: *Picking Sally up from school.*

What I observed about my child: *Sally collapsed in sobs in the car. She begged me to talk to her teacher so she wouldn't have to give reports in class. When I asked how it went, she said she could barely talk and now everyone thinks she's a stupid baby. She refused to go to the next soccer game, because her classmates are on the team, and she is too embarrassed.*

How I responded: *I asked Sally specifics about the report and reassured her it probably was better than she thought. She angrily replied that I didn't know what I was talking about. I tried to cheer her up and reason with her, but she would have none of it.*

Fear thermometer number: *9*

I suggest monitoring your child every day for at least a week. You will find a blank Parent Monitoring Worksheet online in appendix A (http://www.newharbinger.com/39539). Here are some ways to focus your monitoring efforts:

- Make a mental list of the times in your child's day that you want to observe: waking up, having breakfast, dressing and grooming, leaving for school, doing homework, eating dinner, going to bed, and sleeping through the night.
- Focus observation on times or activities during which you have noticed your child exhibit anxiety or avoidance behaviors.
- Consider feedback you have received from teachers, other parents, or friends about situations in which your child became distressed.
- Brainstorm with your child's other parent or caregiver regarding situations he or she may have observed your child experience distress.
- Write down what you learn. Rather than chronicling every detail, focus on the most frequent and most distressing situations.
- Take quick notes during the day and then enter them on the worksheet at the end of the day (or at a time convenient to you).

This can be done in as little as five to ten minutes per day.

Throughout monitoring, I suggest you adopt a matter-of-fact attitude. Keep your observations devoid of judgmental terms. Don't write, "John was at the supermarket and freaked out." Instead, stick to the facts and record them as specifically and succinctly as possible: "At the supermarket, John refused to touch the shopping cart. He kept his hands in his pockets, seemed irritable, and repeatedly asked when we could leave. When I realized I had forgotten the ground beef for tomorrow's spaghetti, he became angry. I asked him to run and grab a pound of beef. He tried to convince me to come back on my own the next day. He refused to get the meat. I had to get it myself." Report events in the same manner an impartial observer might use to record your child's behavior. This businesslike, benign perspective sets the tone for the treatment to come.

Monitoring does not have to be a secret. Be open with your child about this process. A simple and direct explanation, such as "I'm gathering information so we can help you worry less," is usually sufficient.

Some children choose to maintain their own worksheets. If your child wants to do this, feel free to encourage it. In my experience, children as young as eleven or twelve are capable of self-monitoring; however, you know your child's abilities, so let that rather than age be your guide. You will find a Child Monitoring Worksheet in appendix B (h ttp://www.newharbinger.com/39539). Every bit of information can prove useful when developing a treatment plan. Never, however, force or coerce a child into self-monitoring.

If your child objects to your monitoring his behavior, explain that this is a useful step in helping him feel better. Ask him what he thinks will happen if you monitor his anxious responses. Perhaps he fears your increased focus on his anxiety will cause him to spend more time thinking about and feeling that anxiety. Refer to the worry hill and explain how every step up the hill brings him closer to coasting down the other side, where he will feel less worried.

Downward Arrow Technique

After you have recorded your observations for a week on your Parent Monitoring Worksheet, you should be able to see patterns in your child's behavior. You will notice that the anxiety behaviors are manifesting in certain types of situations. Now you can sit down with your child and begin to discern what she specifically fears about the situation.

The downward arrow technique guides you through a series of questions about what your child thinks will happen when he can't avoid a given trigger situation. This allows you to zero in on the consequence your child fears the most in that situation. Each arrow represents one step closer to the true underlying cause of anxiety. A blank Downward Arrow Worksheet you can complete with your child is included in appendix C (http://www.newharbinger.com/39539).

As you use the downward arrow technique with your child, review table 2, which provides examples of the relationship between trigger situations and feared consequences. This gives you an idea of what you may find for a range of situations.

**TABLE 2. Examples of Common Triggers
and Feared Consequences**

Situation	Feared Consequence
Raise hand in class	I will get the answer wrong, stumble on my words or go blank, and kids will think I'm stupid or weird.
Use public restroom	I will touch germs or other people's body fluids and get sick or worry about having yucky stuff on me.
Pack backpack for school	I will forget something important, and my grades will suffer.
Parents go out and child has a new sitter	Something bad will happen, and my parents won't come home. I might not feel well and need Mom to help me.
Take the school bus	I get really nervous. I might throw up. If I throw up, kids will think I'm gross and weird.
Make small talk with an acquaintance	I will have nothing to say or stumble over my words, and there will be awkward silences. Other kids will think I'm stupid and not like me anymore.
Ride elevators	The elevator will break. I will be stuck and get so scared I will shake and feel like I'm dying or having a heart attack.
Items are out of order	I am so bothered seeing things out of order that I won't be able to do anything else or relax until I put them in the correct order.
Encounter a big dog	The dog will bite me, lick me, or jump up on me.

The trick when using the downward arrow technique is to be persistent and to continue asking questions until you reach your child's most feared consequence. I will walk you through this process with examples that show step-by-step how to use the technique with your child. Each example starts with a dialogue in which the parent asks the child what he fears will happen (the feared consequence) in a trigger situation. This is followed by the Downward Arrow Worksheet that the parent filled out. I have added notes to the dialogue to highlight the strategies you can use when employing this technique. In each dialogue, I refer to the mother or father as "parent" to reinforce the idea that either parent can take this role.

Eight-Year-Old John

Parent: John, I noticed you didn't want to touch the cart while we were in the grocery store, and you looked worried. So I wanted to ask you something: What will happen when you touch the cart?

John: I don't know.

Parent: I understand you haven't thought about this. But let's just pretend. What do you think might happen if you did touch the cart? (*John remains silent.*) I know you may not know right now, but let's try to figure this out.

John: I don't know, Mom. How?

Parent: Well, I learned about some ways that might help us figure it out. Let me ask you a question, John. What will happen if you touch the cart?

John: I don't know.

[You may need to pose your questions many times. Do not be discouraged.]

Parent: Okay, you read cartoons. You know the thought bubbles that show what a character is thinking? Picture yourself in a cartoon, touching a shopping cart. What might the words be in the bubble above you?

John: I don't know.

[Here you might offer examples, one at a time.]

Parent: Well, some people might be worried about touching germs.

John: Yeah, I don't want to touch the germs.

Parent: I see. What would happen if you did touch the germs, and you knew there were germs on your hands?

John: It would just be yucky. I might get sick.

Parent: What do you mean "get sick"?

John: I might catch a cold or the flu.

[At this point, you might want to restate what your child has told you so far.]

Parent: Okay, John. What you've told me is you don't want to touch the shopping cart because you might touch germs and then catch a cold or the flu. I wonder ... what would happen if you caught a cold or the flu?

John: If I got a cold, my nose would be stopped up.

Parent: I see. And what would happen if your nose got stopped up?

John: Then it would be hard for me to breathe.

Parent: Yeah, that's no fun. You might have to blow your nose a lot and stuff. But what will happen if you have trouble breathing?

John: I worry I'd stop breathing at night.

Parent: Wow, that's a big worry. So tell me what might happen if you stopped breathing at night?

John: I could die.

John's mother used this conversation to fill out a Downward Arrow Worksheet (figure 3).

Situation:

Touching a grocery store shopping cart

What will happen in this situation?

Other people's germs are all over the cart.

What will happen if...*people's germs are all over the carts?*

I might catch a cold or the flu.

What will happen if...*you catch a cold or flu?*

I will feel terrible and get all stuffed up.

What will happen if...*you feel terrible and get all stuffed up?*

I won't be able to breathe at night.

What will happen if...*you are unable to breathe at night?*

I might die in my sleep.

Figure 3. Downward Arrow Worksheet
(Completed by John's Parent)

We have now established the fear structure for eight-year-old John. He doesn't fear shopping carts per se; he fears that the germs on the cart will make him sick, prevent him from breathing at night, and lead to death. This is a very frightening position to be in for a young child. You can see that arriving at the final feared consequence took persistent questioning. It never hurts to ask the next arrow question, even if it seems self-evident or too scary. Ask and ask and ask. You may be surprised at what you find. In this case, John's parents also learned that many other situations, such as using public restrooms and touching other things in public places, trigger his fears of being contaminated by germs and becoming so ill he can't breathe.

The following two examples underscore why it is crucial not to rely on your own assumptions about what your child fears about a particular situation. Children may manifest similar behaviors, but their fear structures may be quite different.

Haley and Camilla are twelve years old and score well on tests and homework and generally receive good grades. However, both refuse to speak in class, will not raise their hands to answer questions, and sit at the back of the classroom whenever possible. In both cases, their teachers have alerted the parents to the problem, which has worsened over the school year. At face value, you might assume these girls share a common problem, but the downward arrow discussion reveals each child's individual fear structure.

Twelve-Year-Old Haley

Parent: Haley, as you know, we had our parent-teacher conference yesterday, and one of the issues that keeps coming up is that your teacher would like you to participate more in class.

Haley: (Shrugging) I don't know, Dad. I just don't have anything to say.

Parent: You don't have anything to say? Really? Let's look at this together. What were you studying in history?

[Here is an opportunity to examine the evidence—an approach particularly useful with an older child.]

Haley: The Aztecs.

Parent: Okay. Your teacher probably asked questions. Do you remember what she asked?

Haley: Yeah, she asked dumb stuff, like "Who is the Aztec sun god?"

Parent: Why is that a dumb question?

Haley: Everyone knows that.

Parent: And it sounds like you knew, too, so you could have answered. But you decided not to. What about English class? You told me how much you're enjoying *The Outsiders* and like Ponyboy. Did your teacher ask any questions about the book?

Haley: Yeah, she did.

Parent: And did you know the answer?

Haley: Yeah.

Parent: Okay, this sounds similar to what happened in history. You didn't want to raise your hand in either class?

Haley: Hmm.

Parent: So it seems you do have something to share. Maybe we can figure out what is getting in the way of your sharing.

[Together you and your child have examined the evidence and debunked the assertion she has nothing to say. Now you can continue with the downward arrow.]

Parent: What do you think will happen if you talk in front of a class?

Haley: I don't know.

Parent: Well, picture yourself in English. If you know the answer to a question—what do you think will happen if you raise your hand?

Haley: When I get nervous, my voice might shake.

Parent: Good for you for discovering that! If you give an answer and your voice shakes, what will happen?

Haley: Everyone will know I'm nervous about answering an easy question.

Parent: Okay, that's interesting. Let's say you answer the question and your voice shakes, and you know everyone knows you're nervous. What will happen then?

Haley: I don't know. I just don't want people to notice I'm nervous.

Parent: I understand it's uncomfortable to be nervous in front of people, but what will happen? Are you worried they won't think you're smart or something?

Haley: Most kids know I'm smart.

Parent: So then, what would be so bad about your voice shaking and the other kids knowing you're nervous?

[Remember that you need to repeat yourself with this technique.]

Haley: They might think I'm weird.

Parent: That's really interesting. Let's take it one step further.

Haley: You're going to ask me what will happen if kids think I'm weird!

Parent: You're so perceptive, Haley! So...?

Haley: If other kids think I'm weird, they won't like me and won't want to be my friend anymore.

Parent: Good job, Haley! I think this will help us come up with a plan so you can worry a little less about people thinking you're weird. Let's get a snack, shall we?

Haley's father filled out a Downward Arrow Worksheet after this conversation (figure 4). Notice how accurately each answer summarizes what Haley described as her expected consequences.

Situation:

Raising my hand and answering a question in front of the class.

What will happen in this situation?

I might get nervous, and my voice might shake.

What will happen if..._you get nervous and your voice shakes?_

Other kids will know I am nervous.

What will happen if..._kids see and know you are nervous?_

They will think I'm weird for getting nervous.

What will happen if..._kids think you are weird because you seem nervous?_

They won't like me anymore.

What will happen if...

Figure 4. Downward Arrow Worksheet
(Completed by Haley's Parent)

Twelve-Year-Old Camilla

Camilla manifests similar behaviors to those of Haley; however, the following conversation shows that her anxiety has a different source.

Parent: Camilla, as you know, we met with your teacher yesterday, and she's worried about your reluctance to participate in class. Your work is excellent, but you are losing participation points and that could affect your grade.

Camilla: What? I'm losing points?

Parent: Well, our real concern isn't so much your grade, but your reluctance to speak. Is there a reason you choose not to participate?

Camilla: Gosh, Mom, I don't know. I just get so nervous.

Parent: Can I ask you a couple questions that might allow us to figure this out and to help you with it?

Camilla: Okay, if you think it will help. [Notice that Camilla is somewhat more cooperative than Haley.]

Parent: Think of a time in class this past week when you could have raised your hand but chose not to.

Camilla: All right.

Parent: What were you thinking when you decided not to raise your hand?

Camilla: Usually I'm thinking that I'm not 100 percent sure my answer is right.

Parent: Let's say you raised your hand even though you were only 80 percent sure. What would happen then?

Camilla: I might give the wrong answer in front of everyone.

Parent: That's good, Camilla: I'm beginning to understand. Let's say you gave an answer, and it was wrong—what would happen then?

[This question can provoke an anxious reaction. Your child might look tearful or upset.]

Camilla: Well, I'm smart, and most kids expect me to get the answers right.

Parent: I understand, but what if you didn't get the answer right one time? What would happen? Are you worried you'd be embarrassed, or is there something else that bugs you?

Camilla: I think I'm more upset about getting it wrong for myself. I don't like to get anything wrong. I usually check all my answers before I turn anything in. So if I'm not sure I'm right, I could get the answer wrong, and I'd hate that!

Parent: It sounds like what scares you is not being sure you have the right answer, and you can't check to be sure if you're on the spot in class.

Camilla: That's right. It makes me nervous if I don't know for sure I've got it right.

Parent: I'm impressed! Look at how much we're learning about you! So, it sounds like you only take a shot at answering a question when you are 100 percent sure you know the answer. That kind of makes me sad, because you're in school to learn. You aren't expected to know everything already. That must be hard for you.

Camilla: I know I worry more than I should. I know my teacher won't care if I get a question wrong. She has told me a million times that it's the effort that is most important, but I just get scared I'll be wrong. Even when she calls on me personally, I get too nervous to answer.

Parent: Camilla, I'm proud of you for talking to me about this, and I know I'm sounding a little like a broken record, but what is it about not being sure you have the right answer that scares you? Let's pretend you were not sure of an answer but decided to take the risk and give the answer anyway, and it turned out your answer was wrong.

Camilla: The thought of it scares me. I hate being wrong! I'd rather not take the risk at all.

Parent: I get that, but let's pretend you did. What would the thought bubble above your head say?

Camilla: It would say, "Camilla, if you get it wrong, Miss Ace will give you a bad grade."

Parent: Okay, I don't think Miss Ace would give you a bad grade for missing one answer—she's even told you that many times—but what if you do miss an answer and get a bad grade? What will happen then?

Camilla: Then my whole grade for the class will be lower.

Parent: Okay, what will happen if your whole grade is lower?

Camilla: I want all As. You know that!

Parent: I do know that, but just try to answer my questions so we can get to the bottom of these worries.

Camilla: Well, if my grades aren't good, I won't get into a good college. You know I really want to go to Harvard like you did. If I get a bad grade, I can't get into Harvard.

Parent: I didn't know you worried about not being able to get into Harvard. That's a long way off.

Camilla: Well, my grades count now for high school. If my grades aren't good enough, I won't get into one of the best high schools, and then I won't get into Harvard.

Parent: Okay, one last question. What will happen if you don't get into Harvard?

Camilla: Then I won't get a good job I really like. I might end up poor and super unhappy. I'd always regret I didn't push myself harder to get perfect grades.

[This last step probably would need to be broken down, as in previous steps.]

Parent: Camilla, good work. I'm learning how we might be able to work on these fears so you don't worry so much and so it doesn't get in the way of your schoolwork. Let's talk about it more another day.

Camilla: Okay, Mom. That sounds good. I feel kind of silly because I know I shouldn't be so worried, but I am.

Camilla's mother filled out the Downward Arrow Worksheet in figure 5. If you compare this worksheet and the one for Haley, you can see how their answers diverge from the first arrow, indicating that each child has a different anxiety issue.

Applying the Downward Arrow Technique

This technique can cause some discomfort and anxiety, because your child will have to face his fear in his mind, without being in the real-time trigger situation. Ideally, you can have this conversation following an anxiety-provoking incident. Although you do not want to attempt this discussion in the heat of the moment, while your child is still agitated, it is best to apply downward arrow while the situation is still fresh in both your minds.

Engaging in the downward arrow analysis can have a therapeutic effect on its own. Children are sometimes surprised to discuss their fears in this depth—and to see, on paper, the irrational nature of their fears. They likely have been avoiding thinking about them, and so simply bringing them to light can have a positive effect. An analogy I like to use with parents and children is the "monster during the night." In the darkness, the child might imagine a monster lurking in the room, but in the light of day, the feared object is seen to be a pile of laundry. The same is true of fear. Shedding light on fears through the downward arrow technique can frequently provide a child with a much more objective perspective on her anxiety.

The primary purpose of the downward arrow technique, however, is to assess your child's fear structure. Resist any temptation to use this technique to prove to her how irrational her feared consequences are. That would be counterproductive. You and your child will use this information about the structure of her fears to move on to the next steps in this program, such as correcting thinking errors through smart talk or doing exposures.

Situation:

Raising my hand and answering a question in front of the class

What will happen in this situation?

I might get the answer wrong. I need to be 100% sure I've got the right answer before I'll say it in front of the class.

What will happen if..._you aren't 100% sure you've got the right answer. Everyone expects me to get things right, and I hate getting anything wrong!_

What will happen if..._you get something wrong?_

I'll be so disappointed and stressed.

What will happen if..._you're disappointed and stressed?_

It feels terrible, and then I won't get into a good college or get a good job.

What will happen if..._you don't get into a good college?_

I'll have a terrible life and will never be happy.

Figure 5. Downward Arrow Worksheet (Completed by Camilla's Parent)

A Few Last Words of Advice and Caution

Your child may repeatedly refuse to discuss anxiety in any way. Don't let being rebuffed discourage you. You may have to wait for the proper opening for your child to be able and willing to verbalize his feelings.

You may also find you have an emotional reaction of your own to what your child uncovers. The fear structures of anxious children can seem alarming, sinister, weird, or frustratingly silly. Try not to read too much into what your child tells you. For example, if your child worries about hurting someone by accident or can't get a gruesome image out of his mind, don't assume he has excessive anger or violent tendencies. Maintain a nonjudgmental, curious attitude. If you appear apprehensive, your child may sense this and not trust you with the process. So be supportive and praise your child as he reveals his fears. Go at a pace that seems relatively comfortable for your child. If your child seems overwhelmed at any given moment, step back or take a break, but be sure to get back to the process.

Remember that, as a parent, you are not—and should not expect yourself to be—a clinician or diagnostician. You can help your child just by using the information in this book. Having a clear understanding about your child's fear structure is one of the first steps in this program. Once you have it, you can begin to work with your child to conquer those fears. Knowledge of your child's fears will also be important as you plan exposure work.

Finally, if you feel too apprehensive or uncomfortable with the content of your child's fears, I suggest you contact a CBT clinician who is experienced in treating children with anxiety disorders. Do read the entire book, however, because what you learn here will help you find effective support for your child.

SUMMARY: What Did You Learn from This Chapter?

- Processes that are helpful for identifying triggers and their associated fear structures include monitoring and the downward arrow technique.

- Anxiety is not usually a free-floating feeling; something specific triggers a fear response in your child.
- You can determine what triggers your child's fears by noticing the situations in which your child becomes distressed, worried, or avoidant.
- Monitoring involves observing the situations in which your child experiences anxiety and noting how you respond to your child in these situations.
- To start, monitor your child every day for at least a week.
- The downward arrow technique allows you and your child to establish his or her fear structure and recognize the consequences for each trigger situation.
- Using the downward arrow analysis can have a therapeutic effect on its own, but its main purpose is to determine your child's fear structure.

CHAPTER 5

Stop Feeding Your Child's Fear

During times of need, all healthy children seek the comfort, guidance, and protection a parent can provide. Anxious children experience higher levels of distress than do other children, and therefore tend to rely more heavily on their parents when their fears are triggered. I meet parents of anxious children every day who tell me about the myriad manners in which they try to comfort their anxious children. They tell me it is exhausting, stressful, and disruptive to their family's day-to-day lives. Sometimes parents feel so helpless and stressed about their child's anxiety and their attempts to quell it that they become angry with their child and feel worse still.

Many parents I have worked with exhaust themselves reassuring or rationalizing with their child, trying to convince him that his fears are irrational. Out of desperation, they will help him avoid situations that trigger anxiety, even though avoidance reinforces his fears. They do this because they have no other effective means of helping to reduce distress. Indeed, some parents have told me that even psychiatrists, behavioral pediatricians, psychologists, and other mental health professionals recommended some form of avoidance or distraction to alleviate a child's distress. These recommendations are counterproductive and are not based on sound or current scientific evidence.

Many parents whose children have anxiety about sleeping alone, for example, develop elaborate bedtime rituals—playing soft music, providing special relaxation mattress pads, or promising multiple check-ins—or they allow the child to sleep with them or on the floor in a sleeping bag. Many parents of older children tell me their adolescent texts them excessively, seeking or demanding reassurance that all is well. Some parents, out of desperation, allow children to miss school, thinking that a "mental health day" could provide relief and at least can't do any harm.

Parents can fall easily into a pattern. Sometimes, after years of interceding for an anxious child, parents lose perspective about the scope and impact of their own behaviors. Even many highly educated, intelligent, and well-meaning parents can develop numerous extreme behaviors in response to an anxious child. These behaviors that parents adopt are referred to by scientists as "parental accommodations." Parental accommodation is an extensively studied and well-documented phenomenon in families with children suffering from anxiety disorders, and the higher the level of parental accommodation, the poorer the treatment outcome tends to be. These studies also show that the more parents accommodate to an anxious child, the more severe the child's anxiety symptoms are (Garcia et al. 2010; Merlo et al. 2009). Researchers at Yale are now studying whether reducing a parent's accommodating behaviors could be effective enough to serve as the sole treatment for a child with anxiety.

My experiences mirror the scientific data. In fact, most well-intentioned parents who consult with me unintentionally feed their child's problems by accommodating to their child's fears. This is why I work closely with them to gradually reduce their accommodating behaviors. With the help of this book, you too will learn how to reduce your level of accommodation. You can play a crucial role in your child's recovery by addressing your own behavior. This chapter explains what these accommodating behaviors are and how to reduce your use of them.

We'll talk about how you as a parent can alter your behaviors so you can regain control over some of the factors that contribute to your child's anxiety issues. Don't take this as a criticism of your parenting or anything of the sort. It's about rationally identifying the factors that contribute to your child's anxiety and then correcting course. To start, we will look at avoidance and safety behaviors, and then I will discuss the steps you can follow to reduce your use of them with your child.

First, however, I want to give you a little more terminology and a note about obsessive-compulsive disorder (OCD). In CBT, we refer to accommodating behaviors that accompany anxiety problems as "avoidance and safety behaviors." An avoidance behavior is any attempt to avoid being in or thinking about a situation that triggers fear. Safety behaviors are things a person does (through actions or thoughts) to make suffering the feared consequence of being in a trigger situation less likely. People with OCD take accommodating behaviors one step further and develop rituals to help them mitigate what they fear. Just as parents of anxious children can become enmeshed with their child's avoidance and safety behaviors, parents with children who have OCD often engage with their child in compulsions and rituals. For example, if your child has contamination obsessions, you might participate in rituals such as providing hand sanitizers, wiping off cutlery at a restaurant, and providing excessive reassurance that a surface is clean. If you suspect your child has OCD, please don't skip ahead to chapters 10 and 11. Keep reading, because there are more similarities than differences regarding how to help your child conquer OCD and other anxiety issues.

Avoidance Behaviors

Avoidance is typically one of the first strategies a child will use when confronted with a situation that triggers anxiety. It can be an instinctive response for many parents as well. Your child fears dogs; you decide to help your child by keeping him away from dogs. Problem solved. Or so you may think.

In the short run, avoidance works. If a child is never in a situation that could trigger his anxiety, the anxiety will not be triggered. Unfortunately, though, avoidance is harmful in the long run. Avoidance feeds your child's fears by training his brain that the feared situation is indeed something to fear. Each time he avoids a situation, his brain learns to be more afraid of that kind of situation. Moreover, avoidance makes it impossible for him to learn to conquer that fear. Avoidance breeds more avoidance and can generalize to other situations, causing your child to be increasingly fearful. Agoraphobia provides an example of how this works. Agoraphobia is a type of panic disorder in which a person experiences panic attacks and fears having additional episodes. Panic attacks are often first triggered in a specific situation. For example, perhaps your child is climbing the slide at the park and experiences a panic attack. She then feels a need to avoid the park in order to be safe from further panic episodes. Later, however, in a different situation—perhaps a library visit—another attack occurs. She now believes both the park and the library must be avoided—and maybe soon the grocery store as well. Ultimately, she avoids exposure to so many situations that she becomes housebound, because home is perceived as the only place that is safe and won't set off an attack.

Avoidance thus reinforces your child's fear and actually causes it to grow and spread. This means you need to stop condoning the avoidance strategy. What you may think of as helping her is actually hindering. For this reason, Michael Tompkins (2013), a leading anxiety disorder expert, speaks about reducing avoidance as the primary way to conquer all fear and anxiety.

Safety Behaviors

Safety behaviors are strategies both children and parents adopt to make it less likely the child will experience the feared consequence of being in a trigger situation. For instance, suppose your child fears vomiting. Together, you and your child craft a specific diet you believe will prevent him from vomiting. This is a safety behavior in which both of you participate. Although it may seem practical, this safety behavior ultimately will cause his fear of vomiting to increase instead of abate.

Countless safety behaviors can be used both independently and with other important people in your child's life. In my experience, many parents of anxious children contribute to their child's safety behaviors in some way and sometimes even develop their own behaviors to complement or reinforce those safety behaviors. Suppose your child receives an invitation to a playdate. Concerned about her fear of dogs, you call ahead to confirm that the family does not have dogs before approving the playdate. In this example, you build your child's social life around the fear structure. You may believe you are helping—and in the short term, you are solving the problem—but each time you engage in such behaviors, you contribute to your child's anxiety about the situation and make it less likely she will overcome her fear.

Providing excessive reassurance to an anxious child is another common yet detrimental way parents try to provide safety in the face of a child's anxiety. Consider the following exchange between a mother and child who fears vomiting:

Child: Will that apple make me throw up, Mommy?

Parent: That apple is fine, honey. It won't make you sick.

Although this may appear to be an innocuous answer on the parent's part, the child is getting the message that all food has to be cleared through the parent, and it's not safe to eat something unless the danger has been eliminated. The next time the child sits down to eat, he is similarly anxious. Each time, he demands reassurance, because all foods trigger the fear response: "Mom, is this banana going to make me sick?" "What about the sandwich? Is it okay?" By providing excessive reassurance at each query, the parent unknowingly enables the child's fear and prevents him from learning to be less fearful of food.

At this point, I'm sure you are thinking, *Well, how am I supposed to respond to my child so I don't contribute to his anxiety?* Next we will talk about the steps you can take to change your behaviors.

Stopping Both Avoidance and Safety Behaviors

Here I outline how you can stop engaging in avoidance and safety behaviors with your child.

Step 1. Identify Your Behaviors

Start by determining how you may be reinforcing your child's anxiety. Table 3 lists some of the behaviors parents engage in that aid and abet a child's fears. Do you identify with any of these counterproductive behaviors?

TABLE 3. Common Behaviors by Parents

Avoidance Behaviors	Safety Behaviors
Allowing your child to avoid certain locations, such as parks, grocery stores, movie theaters	Providing excessive reassurance to your child in situations she fears
Making excuses for your child to avoid sleepovers or playdates	Rationalizing and explaining to your child why his fears are irrational
Avoiding watching the news or discussing current events that trigger your child's fears	Making changes in your child's schedule to accommodate her fears
Allowing your child to leave a situation if he feels anxious	Serving only foods your child is comfortable with or frequenting only specific "safe" restaurants

To help you identify your behaviors, return to the Parent Monitoring Worksheet you completed in chapter 4. Observe the patterns in your behaviors and responses to your child's anxious reactions. Next, begin the process of completing the Avoidance and Safety Behaviors I Do with My Child Worksheet. A blank worksheet can be found in appendix D (http://www.newh arbinger.com/39539). Table 4 shows what Haley's father wrote on his worksheet.

TABLE 4. Avoidance and Safety Behaviors I Do with
My Child Worksheet (by Haley's Father)

Situation	Avoidance and Safety Behavior
Mother of Haley's friend calls to arrange a playdate or sleepover.	I make excuses for Haley so she doesn't feel pressured to go. I try to convince Haley to go and reassure her it will be fine and she'll have lots of fun.
Haley's sister Marie has friends over.	I allow Haley to eat dinner in her room to avoid Marie's friends. I tell Marie and her friends that Haley has a school project and needs to work alone in her room.
Haley has an oral report.	I reassure her repeatedly. I explain to her why she shouldn't worry. I give her chamomile tea.

Step 2. Develop a Plan to Reduce Your Participation

You will need to come up with a plan to gradually relinquish your participation in avoidance and safety behaviors. The more your child has relied upon you for these behaviors, the more challenging it will be for you and your child to change course. Your child's fear thermometer ratings will rise when he sees you begin to pull back. To mitigate distress, the plan you come up with should gradually reduce your participation in these behaviors.

Start by taking the list you completed in the previous step and find a quiet time to dialogue with your child about what you've learned. Your child is already familiar with the process involved in conquering his fears, so this discussion should not seem like it's coming out of the blue. Explain that some of the ways you respond when your child is worried are not helping him. In fact, some of these responses may interfere with his ability to conquer his anxiety.

With your list in hand, go through each avoidance and safety behavior you do with your child and ask him, "How high would your fear thermometer rating be if I did not do this behavior in this situation?" For example, note the fear thermometer estimates Haley gives when asked how hard it would be for her to be in the trigger situation if her father refrains from engaging in each behavior. Haley provides a range for each fear rating because she is giving an estimate and because her rating will vary depending on the nature of the situation in which her father does that behavior. Thus, for example, her fear rating would be between a 2 and a 4 when her father provides reassurance and rationalizes.

- Providing reassurance and rationalize (2–4)
- Allowing her to avoid situations (5–9)
- Making excuses for her so she can avoid fearful situations (2–6)

Reviewing Haley's list shows us that her father no longer giving reassurance and rationalization is where they should start, as it will cause Haley the smallest rise in her fear thermometer ratings. Haley and her father should agree that he will stop reassuring her and will resist the urge to explain to Haley why she shouldn't be so worried in specific situations.

Even though your child will not be doing formal exposures yet, reducing avoidance and safety behaviors obviously leads to some degree of exposure and, hence, distress. As in

Haley's case, if your child first relinquishes those behaviors that cause her the least anxiety, the process will be more tolerable. Baby steps like these also increase your child's willingness to participate in the program.

Step 3. Change Your Behavior

When you and your child have identified the first behavior you are going to stop, your goal is to refrain from engaging in that behavior in the agreed-upon situations going forward. Your child will invariably experience some days that are harder than others and may beg you to reinstate that behavior. Your job is to resist that temptation, especially if your child becomes distressed when he has to do without your accommodation. The following are some suggestions to help you and your child reach this goal.

First, before you make real-life changes, do a trial run with your child to see how things will go. Troubleshooting ahead of time like this is especially helpful if you anticipate that you or your child may struggle with stopping a particular avoidance or safety behavior. Even if you think this first step will be relatively easy, it's always best to be prepared by practicing beforehand. Practice and repetition are a big part the process of conquering anxiety. You and your child will learn something new each time you practice.

The best way to troubleshoot is to pretend with your child that you are in a trigger situation that typically leads to your participation in the target safety or avoidance behavior. In preparation, consider the following questions:

- What will happen when my child and I stop engaging in these behaviors?
- What will I say to my child instead of giving reassurance?
- How will I handle seeing my child in distress?
- How can I help my child in these moments?
- What can my child do to as self-help when things get difficult?

You and your child will want to identify and practice possible solutions for challenges that may arise. For this, look to the basic tools you and your child have already learned—nicknaming the fear and reading the fear thermometer—and possibly other strategies that you'll learn later in this book, such as smart talk (chapter 7) or playing team tag with your child's other parent.

Here is a conversation between Haley and her father, which builds on their earlier dialogue, as they troubleshoot ahead of time and then do a trial run of their new behaviors.

Parent: Haley, so we've agreed I won't respond to your worries about other kids not liking you by reassuring you or explaining why you need not be worried, right?

Haley: Right.

Parent: Let's talk about how that could go. Say I pick you up from school, and you're worried Michelle thinks you're weird because she gave you a bad look when you stumbled while answering a math question. And you want to keep explaining what happened so I will reassure you that you didn't do anything weird. What do you think will happen if I don't reassure you?

Haley: I might get annoyed with you.

Parent: Thank you for being honest, sweetheart. What do you think we can do if that happens? Could we use any of the tools we already have?

Haley: I could use my nickname.

Parent: Great idea. Could I ask if Worry Monster is bugging you?

Haley: It would work better if you didn't ask me. Just say, "Worry Monster."

Parent: Good suggestion. This is why we're doing this practice: we want to figure out what works best. Any other ideas for tools that might help us?

Haley: We could use the fear thermometer.

Parent: Excellent. How exactly should we do that? Can I ask what your fear thermometer rating is when you're triggered and want me to reassure you?

Haley: That sounds fine. I'm okay with that.

Parent: So far your suggestions are super! We've got the nickname and the fear thermometer. It's recommended that we practice these a few times.

Haley: How do we do that?

Parent: We can pretend you're triggered and then use the tools. Let's use the situation we just talked about. Pretend I'm picking you up after school, and you're worried about Michelle not liking you. Okay?

Haley: Okay. What do we do?

Parent: Here I am, picking you up. Honey, how was school today?

Haley: Oh, I get it. School was okay, Dad, but I'm really upset because Michelle ignored me after math class. I took a long time to answer a math question Mr. Cook asked me, and I sounded like an idiot! I know she thinks I'm a weirdo now!

Parent: This sounds like Worry Monster. What do you think?

Haley: I guess it could be.

Parent: How about using your nickname? Maybe you could do that silently.

Haley: (*pausing and then smiling*) Okay, I did it.

Parent: What's your fear thermometer rating now?

Haley: About a 4. It was a 6 until Michelle said goodbye to me after school. She still seemed unhappy with me, even though she said bye.

Parent: We did it. I didn't reassure you, and you used two of the tools you have. How do you think it went?

Haley: Pretty well, I guess.

Parent: I think we did a great job. I feel more prepared now. Do you?

Haley: Yes, but I still think it will be hard sometimes.

Parent: I'm sure it will be. But if we keep practicing, it will get easier, and your worries won't bug you as much.

As you troubleshoot with your child, use the tools you are learning in this book, rather than relying on old harmful behaviors or coming up with your own hybrid versions. You may feel so accustomed to relying on safety behaviors that it is hard to try something else. Don't let that stop you. It doesn't matter if you feel awkward or if your child says he doesn't like your new behaviors. The latter is probably a ploy to get you to revert to the old behaviors. Be patient and consistent; you and your child will get the hang of it.

Step 4. Determine the Next Behavior You Will Change

After you and your child feel comfortable doing without the first avoidance or safety behavior you set out to eliminate, return to your Avoidance and Safety Behaviors I Do with My Child Worksheet. Have another discussion with your child and decide together which behavior you want to stop next. Practice and troubleshoot ahead of time, as you did with the first behavior. Continue this process until you have eliminated all of your avoidance and safety behaviors. Make sure you do not go back to engaging in any of the behaviors again. If you do, you will set the stage for relapse.

Tips and Troubleshooting: Strategies to Try If You Get Stuck in the CBT Process

Some parents have a harder time than others relinquishing their participation in avoidance and safety behaviors. Also, some children go to one parent more than the other for these behaviors. In my experience, in traditional families, mothers, rather than fathers, tend to be a child's target when trying to co-opt a parent into engaging in avoidance or safety behaviors. In less traditional families, the dynamics can be different. Typically, though, one parent is more relied upon than the other. We also know that parents who struggle with their own anxiety problems tend to participate in these behaviors with their children more than parents who do not.

Regardless, as a parent, you may instinctively want to provide comfort when your child experiences distress. When you see your child unhappy, you want to jump in and fix it. Here are some strategies to help if you are struggling in this manner. Refer to them whenever you need to get back on track.

Strategy 1: Go Back to the Basics

If you experience difficulty disengaging from your child's fear response, I suggest going back to the toolbox (e.g., monitoring, nicknaming). Refer to the data you collected with the worksheets and use those data to come up with an objective response. Go back to your Parent Monitoring Worksheet and recall how you learned to respond more adaptively. Going back to earlier steps that were effective is always a good strategy. Avail yourself of the tools you are most comfortable with and have experienced to be helpful. Remember that you and your child both need to change behaviors and responses by using these techniques. Returning to the basics can stabilize the program and refocus your efforts.

Strategy 2: Be Consistent

There are countless ways a parent can aid and abet a child—and countless ways a clever child can influence a parent to do so. You, like your child, must work toward altering your behaviors to break the harmful aid-and-abet cycle. Don't underestimate your child's ability to resist giving up avoidance and safety behaviors.

Challenge your child to make steady progress relinquishing each and every behavior, while holding the expectation that she can do so. Be strong and consistent.

If you are unable to remain consistent in your behaviors, your child will struggle. If you occasionally give in, your child will learn that persistent begging, pleading, or becoming angry will accomplish what she wants (your participation in an avoidance or safety behavior). This will lead to more extreme or excessive begging or pleading when you reinstate your efforts to relinquish the behavior. In behavioral theory, we refer to this kind of extreme response as an "extinction burst." Extinction bursts are no fun for anyone. Similarly, lack of consistency on your part can make it harder for your child to cope with a given trigger situation. If your child knows she can lure you into a safety behavior, she will experience more distress in that situation than if she thinks you are unavailable. So doing your part is directly helpful to your child.

Strategy 3: Be Creative

Creativity and flexibility are invaluable as you go about relinquishing your avoidance and safety behaviors. For example, eleven-year-old Matt's mother usually drives him to soccer practice—which Matt fears because he has perfectionist obsessions and worries about making mistakes. If Mom is the one from whom Matt seeks reassurance from via tears, distress, and pleas to miss practice, then perhaps Mom should not drive Matt to practice. Consider sending Matt in a carpool with other teammates or have Dad take him. This behavior shift will likely make it easier for Matt because the person with whom he engages in avoidance and safety behaviors is not present, and thus he will be less likely to have the urge to engage in such behaviors. Of course, Matt will likely have a higher fear thermometer rating when he can't do the safety behaviors, but only temporarily. Once Matt finds it easier to resist the safety behavior, rides with Mom can resume. Matt must continue to resist asking for reassurance, and Mom must agree not to provide it.

Strategy 4: Resist Arguing and Rationalizing

Often parents engage in lengthy dialogues in an attempt to explain to their child why she should not be worried about a particular situation. Your argument is probably rational, but these conversations are counterproductive. They feed your child's fears. For example, let's revisit twelve-year-old Camilla, who exhibited perfectionist behaviors. Camilla was reluctant to participate in class because she feared giving a wrong answer. Her mother felt exasperated and incredulous that her daughter couldn't seem to see reason. She reported saying things such as "Well, Camilla, no one can be right all the time—surely you realize that?" and "Mistakes are just part of learning anything new, right?" The emotions Camilla's mother expressed toward her daughter are understandable. It is tempting to explain to an anxious child why she shouldn't worry, because fear is often highly irrational. These types of rationalizations may comfort your child in the short run, but they only perpetuate fears over the long run. So resist rationalizing. Resist arguing. Instead, begin to use the tools offered in this book.

Strategy 5: Implement a Team Effort

In families with two parents present, the parents need to support each other during this process. As mentioned, making these behavioral modifications can be taxing on both child and parent. If you have done your parent monitoring, you have a clear sense of which parent participates and in which situations. If one parent begins to feel beaten down or unable to abide by the plan, then he or she needs to step back and ask the other parent to take over. Trading off like this is recommended whenever possible, so both parents understand the importance of maintaining a consistent program. Additionally, using your partner as a sounding board can be helpful when you feel yourself weakening or starting to question your decisions. To have your partner affirm your actions and emotions reinforces that this treatment is a team effort.

Strategy 6: Take Five

Remember that when a child is triggered, he tends to believe his fears. There can be a temporary loss of insight, and it can be hard for him to adhere to using the tools and strategies that have been helpful in the past. Allowing a break, during which both parent and child do not talk about the situation, can be helpful.

Before using this strategy with your child, be sure to introduce the "take five" concept. Use your knowledge from chapter 2 about how anxiety works in your child's brain. Remind your child that anxiety comes in spikes and explain that he is experiencing one now. Explain that it will be much more helpful to discuss the situation after the anxiety spike has passed. Be careful not to let this strategy become an avoidance behavior. If your child figures out that he can avoid discussing his anxiety by taking five, then discontinue this strategy.

Strategy 7: Do No Harm

You may struggle with not providing reassurance. I've heard parents argue, "But my goal is to make my child feel safe." Be advised, this should *not* be the goal. Your goal should be to raise a resilient, mentally flexible, and strong person. You must change your mindset if you believe your mission is to shelter your child from all distress.

Just as children begin by taking small steps when they learn to overcome their anxiety, and then building on those steps, so too can parents begin with manageable increments. Although you may feel helpless in the face of your child's anxiety, this book can help you follow the first rule of the Hippocratic oath: do no harm. Do not enable. Do not aid and abet. Do not provide reassurance at every turn. Do not let emotions intrude. Even if initially overwhelmed by the prospect of establishing a corrective plan, begin by ensuring you are not exacerbating the problem.

Remind yourself that you are not being mean if you ask your child to confront her fears. By adhering to the guidelines in these chapters, you are *helping* your child through proven CBT methods. As long as you are careful not to punish or judge or show disappointment, you are not mistreating your child.

SUMMARY: What Did You Learn from This Chapter?

- Avoidance behaviors are attempts to avoid being in or thinking about a particular situation that triggers worry or fear.
- Safety behaviors are strategies that make it less likely the feared consequence of being in a trigger situation occurs.
- You can unintentionally reinforce your child's fears by engaging in behaviors such as allowing avoidance, providing excessive reassurance, rationalizing, assisting

with reliance on safety behaviors, and participating in rituals.

- Identify your participation in such behaviors by reviewing the data you gathered by monitoring your child and your responses to your child.
- Develop and implement a plan to reduce and eventually eliminate your participation in these behaviors.
- Tips to help you relinquish avoidance and safety behaviors include going back to basics, being consistent, being creative, resisting arguments and rationalization, enlisting a team effort, taking five, and doing no harm.

CHAPTER 6

Stop Your Child from Feeding the Fear

Children experiencing high levels of anxiety inevitably develop strategies to reduce their distress that are independent of anything their parents may be doing to protect them. As we discussed in the previous chapter, anxious children often avoid situations that trigger fear. They also frequently co-opt others—especially parents, siblings, friends, and teachers—into providing reassurance, doing things they fear to do themselves, and engaging in other accommodating behaviors. Similarly, anxious children may over-check their work, attempt to distract themselves, ask questions repeatedly, and engage in numerous other strategies and rituals to be certain a feared consequence does not occur.

On the surface, these strategies may appear to help your child cope with her anxiety—and it is true that using such strategies can temporarily alleviate distress. However, just as your responses to your child's anxiety can feed her fears, many of the strategies she develops ultimately feed her fears and prevent her from conquering them. For these reasons, they must be identified, reduced, and—hopefully—eventually eliminated.

There is an analogy I often use with children and parents. Fear is like a tumor that needs a blood supply to stay alive and grow. Avoidance and safety behaviors by both parents and children provide that blood supply to the tumor. Every time a child or parent resists an avoidance or safety behavior, that blood flow is restricted. Over time, the fear is reduced. Just as you work to identify and change your own responses to your child in trigger situations, you must help your child identify the avoidance and safety behaviors he uses independently of you. Let's walk through this process.

Relinquishing Avoidance and Safety Behaviors

There are four steps you can follow to help your child stop engaging in avoidance and safety behaviors.

Step 1. Identify Avoidance and Safety Behaviors

Take some time to brainstorm about your child's behaviors in situations that trigger his fears. If possible, sit down with his other parent and compare thoughts. By this point, you may be adept at identifying these patterns. To be systematic and thorough, review your Parent Monitoring Worksheet from chapter 4 and reference the common avoidance and safety behaviors listed in table 5. Compile a preliminary list of target behaviors. Keep in mind that avoidance and safety behaviors can be idiosyncratic, extreme, and sometimes just plain weird and silly. Don't hesitate to follow up on any behaviors that don't make sense to you or seem crazy.

Now, invite your child to participate in this process. Along with his contributions (I recommend starting with those), use table 5 as a guide to ask him if he engages in any of the most common behaviors. Be sure to pay attention to the unique and personal ways in which your child engages in avoidance and safety behaviors. A straightforward, collaborative approach will be most productive. Simply ask your child directly if he does any of these behaviors when in a trigger situation. Ask even if you have not observed or don't suspect your child engages in a particular safety behavior.

You are likely to find that you and your child are familiar with many of these strategies in one form or another. Be creative, kind, thorough, and matter-of-fact about it. Remember that this is about identifying specific behaviors so your child will feel better, not about finding a fault in your child.

TABLE 5. Common Avoidance and Safety Behaviors in Children

Avoidance: both obvious and subtle, including planning activities to avoid certain situations
Reassurance: questions to parents, Internet research, and other measures to gain certainty that feared consequences will not occur
Distraction tactics: watching television, reading a book, thinking about pleasant things
Checking behaviors: both obvious and subtle, including mental checking done in the child's mind
Leaving or escaping a situation that triggers a fear response
Limiting diet to safe foods
Using a cell phone to call or text a parent when experiencing anxiety or distress
Using a cell phone or computer to avoid social contacts or as a distraction
Sitting or lying down when anxious
Various rituals

Step 2. Complete Worksheet

Now you and your child are ready to complete the Avoidance and Safety Behaviors I Do in Trigger Situations

Worksheet. You can find a blank version in appendix E (http://www.newharbinge r.com/39539). Complete this worksheet with your child in the same way you completed the worksheet identifying your own behaviors.

Plan a quiet time to review the data you and your child have been collecting. Because your child has already learned many important lessons from you, she should be an excellent helper in this effort. This is especially true if she is motivated to conquer her fears.

Start completing the worksheet by listing in the left-hand column all the situations that elicit an anxiety response. Then, for each situation, determine which avoidance and safety behaviors your child uses in that situation. For example, if soccer practice is a trigger situation, the following may be avoidance and safety behaviors:

- Ask if Mom or Dad thinks many dogs will be present today (seeking reassurance)
- Complain about physical ailments to avoid going (avoidance by making an excuse)

- Say I have too much homework (avoidance by making an excuse)
- Tell Mom and Dad that soccer isn't really fun anymore (avoidance by making up an explanation that is inaccurate)
- Position myself on the field as far away from dogs as possible (safety behavior)
- Tell Mom and Dad to make sure everyone with a dog obeys the leash rules at the park (safety behavior)

As you complete the worksheet with your child, you will likely find that she tends to use more than one or a combination of safety or avoidance behaviors in each situation.

Step 3. Use the Fear Thermometer

Go through each behavior used and ask your child how much distress the fear thermometer would show if the behavior were not used. Write this down in the far-right column on the worksheet. Table 6 shows how Haley completed the Avoidance and Safety

Behaviors I Do in Trigger Situations Worksheet. You may also find helpful the following examples showing how Haley's father presented these questions to Haley.

- "Haley, using your fear thermometer, how hard would it be for you to be no more than one minute early to class?"
- "How distressing would it be for you to sit on the school bus without using your headphones?"
- "How high would your fear thermometer rating be if you sat toward the front of the school bus?"

TABLE 6. Avoidance and Safety Behaviors I Do in Trigger Situations Worksheet (by Haley)

Situation	Avoidance and Safety Behavior (fear rating)
Arriving at class	Arrive early, act busy (6)
Participating in class	Hide behind my hair (4) Use very quiet voice (6) Don't raise my hand (8)
Walking between classes, recess, and lunch	Avoid kids I don't know well (9) Pretend not to see someone so I don't have to say hi (4) Use my headphones so kids think I'm busy (3) Rush around so kids don't have a chance to talk to me (4) Go to library at lunch if my good friends are busy (4)
Taking bus to and from school	Use headphones so kids think I'm busy (3) Sit at back of bus, so kids don't notice me (3)

Step 4. Develop a Plan for Your Child to Give Up

Avoidance and Safety Behaviors

Avoidance and safety behaviors strongly reinforce anxiety, so we want to reduce them and hopefully eliminate them as quickly as is possible. There are two methods to help your child do this. One is to develop a plan to help him relinquish behaviors in his daily life that are relatively easy to stop doing, which is explained in this chapter. The other is to help him give up behaviors by using the technique of exposures, which is discussed in detail in chapter 8. It is possible that success with the first method is sufficient, making exposures unnecessary.

Otherwise, simply being able to reduce reliance on avoidance and safety behaviors in his daily life before he starts exposures can expedite the process of doing exposures. Often children rely on a safety or avoidance behavior even when they would not find it hard to relinquish it. Sometimes this happens because fears shift and change, and a safety behavior the child previously relied on is no longer needed. In this case, the child clings to the behavior more out of habit than out of fear. I consider these instances low-hanging fruit—they're the easiest to get rid of.

To devise a plan for your child, use the Avoidance and Safety Behaviors I Do in Trigger Situations Worksheet you just completed. First check the behaviors and fear thermometer ratings and confirm that they remain accurate. Remember, these ratings may get lower as your child goes through the program. Sometimes just looking at the situations and behaviors with objectivity and making a plan can help a child feel less fearful and more motivated to stop these behaviors. You may be pleasantly surprised that your child gives a lower fear thermometer rating than before. Or your child may select a behavior to stop that you thought would be too difficult. Things can change quickly in CBT, and we are always happy about that.

Now identify the lowest fear thermometer ratings—your low-hanging fruit. For example, if we zero in on the lowest fear thermometer ratings on Haley's Avoidance and Safety Behaviors I Do in Trigger Situations Worksheet (table 6), we see these are for refraining from using her headphones and sitting at the back of the school bus. The behaviors you single out at this step may be from more than one situation; that's fine. Create a new list with only the lowest ratings, placing the smallest numbers at the bottom, in the form of a ladder. Note that children who haven't mastered rank order numbering may need extra help with this task.

- Pretend not to see someone so I don't have to say hi (4)
- Rush around so kids don't have a chance to talk to me (4)
- Hide behind my hair in class (4)
- Go to the library at lunch if my good friends are busy (4)
- Use headphones so kids think I'm busy (3)
- Sit at back of the bus so kids don't notice me (3)

When you have formed this new, short list, ask your child which behavior he or she feels most confident about giving up every time he or she is in a situation that triggers the urge to use the behavior. As an example, here is a conversation between Haley and her father about developing a plan to relinquish avoidance and safety behaviors:

Parent: Haley, you are doing such a good job learning how to manage your worries.

Haley: Thanks, Dad.

Parent: Let's figure out which avoidance and safety behaviors you might be willing to give up on a day-to-day basis.

Haley: You mean always?

Parent: That's the idea. You and I know that even though they seem to help you, these behaviors are making your worries stronger.

Haley: Right. So what do we do?

Parent: Let's look at the worksheet we completed together. Remember, I asked you what your fear thermometer ratings would be if you gave up each of those behaviors. (*Haley and her father study the worksheet together.*) Are the ratings still accurate? Would you change any?

Haley: I think not going to the library would have a lower rating now. Yesterday Marsha was playing with some other girls after lunch, and I wanted to go to the library so I wouldn't feel uncomfortable. But I didn't go.

Parent: Wow, Haley, you were really brave. How did it go?

Haley: It wasn't that hard. After a minute, Jasmine came along and showed me a new game. I got into it, so I didn't feel worried at all.

Parent: I'm so proud of you! What would your fear rating be for not going to the library to avoid being with kids you don't know well?

Haley: I think a 3. So, what am I supposed to do now?

Parent: Let's create a new list with just the easiest ratings. Say, the 3s and 4s. And you can add the new rating for going to the library.

Haley: (*making the new list*) Do I have to do all of these?

Parent: No, just the one you think you could stop doing most easily. Which one do you choose?

Haley: It would be pretty easy for me to stop using my headphones on the bus.

Parent: That's a 3. Do you think it would be easier than the other 3s?

Haley: Yeah. It won't be that hard.

Parent: Super! Would you be willing to start that tomorrow?

Haley: Okay, Dad, I can do that.

A good goal is to give up one avoidance and safety behavior per week. It is much better if the task is too easy for your child than if it is too difficult. We want to set your child up for success and to create a plan that is as manageable as possible. The more success your child experiences, the more motivated he will be to follow the plan.

After you and your child have selected the first avoidance and safety behavior to give up, establish a routine for checking in daily with him to see how well he is doing. This is an important aspect of the plan. Don't assume your child will accept your daily check-ins with enthusiasm. Ask if he is okay with you asking once each day. Suggestions about how to reward your child for relinquishing these behaviors, as well as troubleshooting strategies, are described in the following section.

Use Rewards to Motivate Your Child to Stop Avoidance and Safety Behaviors

Rewards were discussed in chapter 3 as a valuable tool. They can be effective for relinquishing avoidance and safety behaviors. In general, this program places a great deal of emphasis on what a child should *not* do. This negative emphasis can be perceived as punitive, even if it is not intended to be so. As I mentioned in earlier chapters, to avoid falling into this pitfall yourself, keep in mind that it is more effective to motivate children through rewards than through punishment. Reward your child frequently. Not only should the reward be individualized to your child's desires, but it should also be sufficient to motivate.

Some youngsters do not need rewards at all. These children are sufficiently motivated by the prospect of gaining control over their fears. But, generally speaking, some type of reward should be included in the treatment plan.

So, let's walk through this process of using rewards to motivate your child. The basic premise is that your child is rewarded for resisting the urge to engage in avoidance and safety behaviors. This strategy is effective in changing many behavioral issues besides anxiety problems.

Step 1. Identify the Target Behavior

You have already identified target behaviors using the Safety and Avoidance Behaviors I Do in Trigger Situations Worksheet.

For example, suppose your child with a contamination obsession has a nightly ritual of questioning you about the meal after she has finished her homework and before dinner time. Her purpose is to make sure everything is clean: "Daddy, did you wash that knife?" "Where did you buy that corn, Dad?" "Mom, is that chicken safe?" Your goal is to eliminate the questioning. Based on your chart, you know your child has rated giving up these questions as 3 on the fear thermometer, making it the easiest behavior to stop on her list.

Step 2. Identify the Target Time

Next, identify a targeted short time. Monitoring can help you find a time, but transition times (e.g., bedtimes, coming home from school) are usually the most effective, because they happen at about the same time every day. Come up with a plan for this period of time, and practice every day. In our example, this could be the ten to fifteen minutes between when your child finishes her homework and when the family sits down for dinner. You decide on a span of time each evening that she can resist the urge to do reassurance-seeking rituals.

The amount of time your child agrees to should be determined by both of you in collaboration. Ask her for a fear thermometer rating for resisting for five minutes, ten minutes, fifteen minutes, and so on. It doesn't matter how short the time span is. What matters is that your child feels highly confident she can succeed. I'd much rather see a task be too easy for a child than too hard. It's easy to make a task harder, but a child can find it difficult to recover from a failed attempt. That being said, even if your child takes on a challenge that was harder than anticipated, finds it was too difficult, and reverts to using the avoidance or safety behavior, your child can learn something from the attempt. Don't be rattled by your child's failure to achieve a goal such as this. Ask her what she learned. Share with her what you may have learned. Then use this information to recalibrate and come up with a plan your child feels more confident attempting.

Step 3. Identify a Reward

Plan a reward your child can earn when he succeeds. It should be a motivating reward (e.g., a special dessert) and must be commensurate with the difficulty of the challenge. For example, eliminating a safety behavior that rates 4 on the fear thermometer will come with a larger reward than the elimination of a behavior that only rates 2. And do not select a reward that would devastate your child if it is not received.

Choose a reward that is both age appropriate and family appropriate—something that reflects your family's values. For young children, the promise of a cookie can be enough to motivate them to eliminate a ritual behavior. For older children, the reward system can be more complex, involving a point system. Your child need not work toward a purely material reward. Many children are motivated by the promise of special time with a parent or by the opportunity to select a family movie for the weekend.

Step 4. Remind Your Child

At the agreed-upon time, you can remind your child, "Okay, John, it's 6:15. Are you ready to resist seeking reassurance until 6:30? Remember, we agreed that your reward for doing this is that you can choose whether we have ice cream or pie for dessert. I bought your favorite ice cream—mint chip—and the blueberry pie you love from Bette's Bakery."

John looks at the clock and nods. Because he knows what to expect and has agreed to the plan, John is likely to comply willingly. Even if he asks for reassurance after 6:30, he gets his reward. However, you should not provide any reassurance, and instead use his nickname and kindly remind him this behavior is not helpful to him: "John, that sounds like Worrybug. Please pass the salt and pepper."

Step 5. Give the Reward

Give your child the reward if he is successful. However, if your child shows resistance to the idea of receiving a reward and persists with the safety behavior, let him miss out on the reward this time—but offer it again next time. He may be testing you. If you have a history of being inconsistent in how you give out rewards or punishments, your child will tend to exert a lot of energy in attempting to get his way, because he will think that if he persists, waits, or throws a tantrum, you will eventually give in.

Step 6. Reevaluate, If Needed

Of course, if the reward plan fails, you must reevaluate the reward. Every child is motivated by different factors. It is your job, as a parent, to put your knowledge and experience to work on behalf of your child and come up with rewards that are good motivators.

Reevaluate your own attitudes toward the giving of rewards. Some parents fear that using rewards is a form of bribery, which they ideologically reject. Others feel that the need to use rewards means they lack effective parenting skills. Yet others worry that giving rewards will spoil their child. In my experience, using rewards does not have any negative side effects. However, if you have these or similar objections to the use of rewards, my advice is to be open to experimenting with these new strategies. Ultimately, you want to do what will help your child overcome anxiety. Any risk of spoiling your child is greatly overshadowed by the benefits of reducing avoidance and safety behaviors.

SUMMARY: What Did You Learn from This Chapter?

- Anxious children develop avoidance and safety behaviors and mental strategies to reduce worry and fear, but these behaviors unintentionally feed their anxiety.
- Common avoidance and safety behaviors children engage in include avoidance, reassurance seeking, checking behaviors, escaping situations that trigger anxiety, throwing temper tantrums or making excuses to avoid or escape trigger situations, engaging in rituals, and requiring parents to participate in safety behaviors.
- Collaborate with your child to identify her avoidance and safety behaviors.
- Develop and implement a plan to help your child relinquish these behaviors, using the worksheets you have completed.

- Use the fear thermometer to help determine the pace at which your child relinquishes these behaviors.
- Use rewards to increase your child's motivation to cease avoidance and safety behaviors.

CHAPTER 7

Correct Thinking Errors with Smart Talk

In the 1960s, Dr. Aaron Beck, the father of modern cognitive therapy, marveled at the myriad "thinking errors" that depressed and anxious individuals make. He noticed that these errors pop up with great frequency, and he termed them "automatic thoughts" because they happen unconsciously, without the individual thinking about them. In his studies and the thousands of clinical trials evidencing the validity of his theory, Beck (1979) also realized that individuals who make thinking errors do not notice that a particular thought doesn't accurately reflect a given situation. Modern cognitive therapy concerns itself largely with correcting thinking errors and has proven to be extremely effective. Some common thinking errors made by anxious children (as well as by adults) are listed in table 7.

Thinking errors are harmful because both children and adults respond to their thoughts and beliefs about situations rather than to the situations themselves. In other words, they process information about imagined situations that do not match the actual situation. And they believe their thinking errors, especially in the moment they are triggered. For this reason, your child's fears may seem irrational or very extreme to you as a parent. Furthermore, thinking errors are unconscious until you identify them and flesh them out. Your child does not recognize that a thought may not be accurate and may dramatically overstate negative outcomes. He or she then experiences the consequences: an accelerated heart rate, butterflies in the stomach, sweaty palms, or feelings of terror.

TABLE 7. Common Thinking Errors

Type of Error	Behavior
Catastrophizing	Assuming the worst-case scenario will occur
Futurizing	Predicting future negative or fearful scenarios
Overprobablizing	Overestimating the probability of negative consequences
Black-and-white thinking	Thinking in extremes—things are perceived as all good or all bad
Mind reading	Assuming you know what someone else is thinking

Parents tend to be good at recognizing when their child is not thinking accurately. In response, they typically attempt to convince the child that his or her fears are not realistic. We have already discussed why providing this type of reassurance is counterproductive. There are, however, cognitive strategies that are effective at correcting thinking errors. This chapter covers one of them: smart talk.

Smart Talk

Smart talk is the tool you will use to help your child correct the thinking errors that contribute to her anxiety. She can use smart talk in trigger situations in daily life as a tool to diminish reliance on avoidance or safety behaviors. By using smart talk over time, her improved thinking becomes as habitual and unconscious as the thinking error was. Furthermore, evidence suggests that using smart talk can help consolidate the new learning achieved through exposures (Craske et al. 2015), though it should not be used during exposures. Ultimately, the goal is to retrain the brain. We humans learn how to fear things much more efficiently than we learn to extinguish those fears, so retraining requires lots of practice.

You likely observed many of the thinking errors your child makes in trigger situations when you used the downward arrow technique in chapter 4. In fact, you may already have done much of the detective work in identifying thinking errors. You and your child will now explore the evidence on which these thinking errors are based and learn how to correct them with smart talk.

Teaching Your Child Smart Talk

Smart talk is a four-step process. First, help your child identify the thinking error. Second, help him evaluate the evidence that supports or refutes the error. Third, help him generate a thought that reflects a more realistic, evidence-based perspective (the smart talk). Finally, guide him in using the corrected thought, the smart talk. Let's look at each of these steps in detail.

Step 1. Identify Thinking Errors

Sit down with your child in a quiet moment and say something like this: "You have been doing a great job working on conquering Worrybug so far. There is another tool I want to teach you that could help even more. This has to do with your thoughts when you are in trigger situations. We already have some ideas about what you think about when you are in trigger situations, but we are going to do a little more detective work. How does that sound?" You may want to give a specific example of something you and your child are working on.

For example, suppose your child has an irrational fear of dogs. When you completed the downward arrow technique regarding this fear, you and your child determined that the ultimate feared consequence of seeing dogs is being attacked and bitten. Now your task is to figure out what thinking errors he makes that contribute to his anxious response when seeing a dog.

You can describe smart talk to you child using the example of a comic strip. Children of any age who find it hard to recognize their thought processes often do so more easily if they imagine their thoughts appearing above their heads in a bubble. I like to use a comic with a blank bubble so children can write their smart talk phrase in the bubble. This helps them get into the habit of using the phrase and adds a little fun to the process. You will find a blank bubble form in appendix F (http://www.newharbinger.com/39539).

As you and your child focus on the particular thoughts she has in a trigger situation, consider if she is making any of the thinking errors listed in table 7:

- Is your child assuming worst-case scenarios (catastrophizing)?
- Does your child focus on fearful scenarios in the future, rather than on what is really happening in the present (futurizing)?
- Does your child assume something terrible will occur every time he or she is in that situation (overprobabilizing)?
- Does your child engage in thoughts that reflect only extremes, without the nuances and shades of gray that occur in real life (black-and-white thinking)?
- Does your child believe that other people think negative things about her (mind reading)?

Write down any of these thinking errors you and your child identify in particular trigger situations. Again, this is not about identifying flaws in your child. Establish an attitude of curiosity about his thoughts and don't be on a mission to correct his thinking. Remain positive and praise any and all suggestions he makes, even if you don't agree with some of them. Identifying the exact thinking error is less important than providing him with an opportunity to consider other ways of looking at a trigger situation.

Many children already sense that their worry thoughts are not accurate, but they can't help but fall back on them during a spike. Thinking errors can be frustrating and confusing, especially to older and more self-aware children (figure 6).

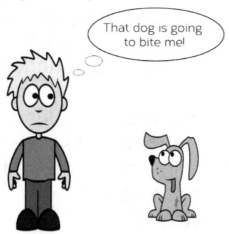

Figure 6. Thinking Error

Step 2. Evaluate the Evidence

An effective way to evaluate the evidence is to ask your child questions about her thoughts so she can consider alternative outcomes. CBT therapists call this process "guided discovery" (Padesky 1993). Guided discovery is similar to the classic tradition of Socratic questioning, in which a teacher asks students a series of questions to stimulate critical thinking and help them reach a conclusion on their own. However, while Socratic questioning can feel a bit like an interrogation, guided discovery should feel like an open-ended, open-minded, collaborative discussion. Gently guide your child to consider alternatives to her fear-based assumptions and beliefs.

Guided discovery entails (1) asking your child a question, (2) listening to your child's response, (3) summarizing what your child told you, and then (4) asking questions that promote an alternative way of thinking about the situation. There are a number of questions that encourage new ways of thinking:

- Does Worrybug's thought always match what happens in real life?
- Does what Worrybug tells you always happen, sometimes happen, or rarely happen? (Using percentages can help your child objectify the situation.)
- Out of ten times when you were in the situation, how many times was Worrybug right? (Be specific, with actual examples.)
- How did you know Worrybug was correct?
- Was it possible that something else happened?
- Has Worrybug ever been wrong?
- Can you think of any times when what you thought was going to happen didn't?

In the following conversation, the father of nine-year-old Henry gently guides him to evaluate any evidence that supports his fear that an off-leash dog will bite him.

Parent: Henry, could we talk a little bit more about what you think will happen if you are around an off-leash dog at soccer practice or the park?

Henry: You already know. I think I'll get bitten!

Parent: I get it: you think that if you see an off-leash dog, it will bite you.

Henry: That's what I said.

Parent: I'm sorry if I sound like a broken record. And I know you don't like talking about this stuff. So I appreciate that you're being patient with me.

Henry: It's okay, Dad. What else do you want to know?

Parent: I want to know if what Worrybug tells you is always right.

Henry: What do you mean?

Parent: Well, for instance, I'm curious if you've ever been around an off-leash dog that didn't bite you?

Henry: Sure, but I'm still scared that one of these days, one will bite me.

Parent: I understand. You haven't been bitten yet, but you're pretty sure a dog will bite you at some time in the future.

Henry: Yeah.

Parent: The Wongs' dog, Duke, sometimes gets out of their yard and wanders over here while you're playing. He did it on Sunday. Do you remember?

Henry: Of course. I was terrified.

Parent: What happened?

Henry: I was so scared that I just froze and waited until Duke left.

Parent: Did Duke bite you?

Henry: No, but he could have.

Parent: He didn't bite you, but he could have. I guess that's true: he could have. Why do you think he didn't on that day?

Henry: I don't know. Maybe he wasn't in the mood.

Parent: So Duke wasn't in a biting mood on Sunday. How did he act when he came up to you?

Henry: He was wagging his tail. And he had a tennis ball in his mouth.

Parent: He had a tennis ball. Why do you think he came up to you with a ball?

Henry: He probably wanted me to throw it. He goes crazy when Mr. Wong throws a ball for him.

Parent: I know! Duke loves playing fetch. Is his excitement about playing fetch what bothers you?

Henry: I hate it. He gets too crazy!

Parent: What could he do if he's so crazy?

Henry: Jump up on me.

Parent: Jump on you, but not bite you?

Henry: Maybe he'd get so crazy that he'd bite me even if I didn't throw the ball for him.

Parent: I guess that's possible. But out of every ten times you've met Duke, how many has he tried to bite you?

Henry: None.

Parent: Do you think it's possible he doesn't bite people?

Henry: I guess so, but you never know. He might.

Parent: So you don't want to risk that.

Henry: Right.

Parent: Sometimes our thoughts make us believe things that don't line up with what actually happens. I think your thoughts about dogs are like that. What do you think?

Henry: Maybe a little, yes.

In this example of guided discovery, we see several of the thinking errors listed in table 7. Henry catastrophized (predicted the dire consequence that a dog would bite him); overprobablized (believed that every time he encountered a dog it would bite him); futurized (predicted that dogs would bite him in the future); and engaged in black-and-white thinking (did not consider all the possible outcomes, such as that a dog might be friendly, might want to play, or might jump up on him). At the end, Henry is moving toward an acknowledgment of his thinking errors.

Step 3. Generate the Smart Talk

The next step is to furnish a rational response, the smart talk. Smart talk should correct the thinking errors your child makes in a straightforward, direct, and simple manner. For example, if your child overestimates the likelihood something will happen, a rational response might be something like "It's possible, but extremely unlikely." Similarly, if you child engages in black-and-white thinking and assumes only extreme outcomes will occur, you can correct that thinking error by saying, "Maybe, but there are lots of other things that can happen."

Keep smart talk short and simple because your child will have to memorize it and use it on the go. Also, be careful not to make smart talk simply a reassurance or pep talk, because that is not effective. For some children, especially younger ones, including the nickname they selected for their fear is helpful and serves not only to correct the thinking error but also to alert them that they are being triggered. This helps children maintain perspective in the face of an anxiety spike.

Here are some general smart talk phrases you and your child can tailor to her particular needs:

- "Just because my friend didn't say hi doesn't mean she doesn't like me."
- "I don't have a crystal ball."

- "It's possible, but lots of other things are more likely to happen."
- "Worrybug, you don't really know how it's going to go."
- "That's catastrophizing! Lots of other things could happen."
- "Nobody's a good mind reader."
- "It's possible, but not likely."

One way to think about generating and using smart talk is to compare it to editing a sentence on your computer. You delete the phrase you wish to change, and you type in the new phrase. Similarly, your child will learn to replace thinking errors with smart talk. If your child assumes the worst possible outcome will always occur when encountering a dog, he can replace the thought *That dog's going to bite me!* with smart talk: *It's possible, but not likely.*

Here is how Henry and his father came up with the smart talk he would use.

Parent: Remember how we talked about your worries that off-leash dogs would bite you, and I asked you about Duke and about other situations in which you worried a dog would bite you but it didn't?

Henry: Yes.

Parent: What did you learn from that discussion?

Henry: That I worry more than I should.

Parent: Let's look at what Worrybug tells you. What does Worrybug say when you see Duke roaming the neighborhood?

Henry: That Duke is going to bite me.

Parent: Right, and has Duke bitten you?

Henry: No.

Parent: So is Worrybug correct so far?

Henry: No, not so far.

Parent: So, that is an example of a thinking error. It makes your fear thermometer rating rise and makes you want to get away from Duke.

Henry: I see what you're saying.

Parent: If we can come up with some smart talk to correct your Worrybug thoughts, you probably won't feel as scared when you see Duke. Also, smart talk will help you resist the urge to do avoidance and safety behaviors, which we learned make your worries bigger and stronger.

Henry: Okay. How do we do it?

Parent: We'd come up with a thought that's more in line with the facts. I can read you this list of smart talk other kids have used. Would that be okay?

Henry: Sure.

Parent: Here they are. (*He reads the entire list of smart talk phrases.*) What do you think?

Henry: There are two I could use: "That's catastrophizing! Lots of other things could happen," and "It's possible, but not likely."

Parent: Excellent! Let's pick the shortest one we think best corrects the thinking errors Worrybug makes you have. Why don't you take a moment and imagine Duke running up to you. Take your fear thermometer rating. Then say each smart talk phrase to yourself and see which one you like the best.

Henry: Okay.

Parent: As Duke is running up to you, what does your fear thermometer say?

Henry: About a 3.

Parent: Great. Now say the first smart talk option. I made it fit your worries and wrote it down on this index card. You can read it if you haven't memorized it. "That's catastrophizing! Lots of other things could happen."

Henry: That kind of helps.

Parent: Good for you! Now let's try the others, and you can decide which smart talk to use when you see off-leash dogs.

Step 4. Practice the Smart Talk

After you and your child have agreed upon the appropriate smart talk, write it down so you, your child, and any other significant caretakers have a record that can be readily referred to (figure 7). Usually, children have one smart talk response for each fear. Your child needs to memorize it and use it exactly as you wrote it together. This is important because, in the heat of an anxious reaction, children often change their smart talk in ways that make it less effective.

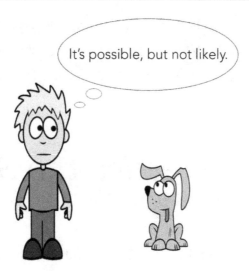

Figure 7. Corrected Thought with Smart Talk

One effective way to practice smart talk is to ask your child to imagine being in the trigger situation, get his fear thermometer rating up, and use the smart talk phrase to interrupt the thinking error. Do this over and over, perhaps ten to fifteen times, until he demonstrates mastery of it. This also provides him with exposure, which is the single most important technique to help him conquer his fears. I discuss exposures further in chapter 8.

Another way to help your child become accustomed to smart talk is to make a game of practicing it. You and your child take turns being Worrybug and Smart Talk (use your child's nickname for "Worrybug"). Ask your child which role she wants to play first. It really doesn't matter who goes first, because the roles will be switched multiple times. The Worrybug role begins the dialogue. Worrybug voices your child's thinking error as if talking to him. In that role, think of all the scary things Worrybug might be telling him. Whoever plays Smart Talk simply responds with the child's smart talk phrase. For Henry, who fears dogs, it might go in part like this:

Worrybug: Henry, you should be really worried about going to the park today. There might be lots of dogs, and one is going to bite you.

Smart Talk: It's possible, but not likely.

This collaborative game invites your child to participate from a position of strength regarding her fears. Be brave, creative, and playful as you play it. Both you and your child should do your best to represent the many facets of Worrybug. You know your child well and know the many ways Worrybug starts in on her. Use this knowledge as you play the game.

Remember, this game involves a mild level of exposure to whatever triggers your child's anxiety. Therefore, it is completely normal for your child to experience an elevation in her fear thermometer rating. This is actually a positive outcome. If you notice your child exhibiting distress, acknowledge it by asking her for a fear thermometer rating, and then continue the game (repeat, repeat, repeat) until she seems more comfortable. The more your child is exposed to the feared situation (even in this indirect manner), the more quickly she will extinguish that fear. Never shy away from what triggers her anxiety. Find a way to address it and move toward it, even if in small increments.

There are a number of ways to help your child during this game:

- Ask what your child's fear thermometer rating is, and then track it as it rises and falls.
- Do many repetitions of the game because every exposure helps your child learn something new.

- Ask your child, "What did you learn by practicing the smart talk?"
- Remind your child not to do any safety behaviors (chapter 5) during the game, because these will interfere with inhibitory learning.
- Encourage your child by giving a reward for playing the game.

Tips and Troubleshooting: Some Words of Caution for Using Smart Talk

A few additional guidelines will ensure your child's work with smart talk is productive.

Smart Talk and Exposures

Smart talk can be used both prior to and after planned exposures, but it should not be used during planned exposures because it can interfere with inhibitory learning.

Smart Talk and OCD

It is vital that your child's problem be clearly identified, as outlined in chapter 4, prior to employing smart talk. Haley and Camilla, the twelve-year-old girls who were having trouble in class, manifested similar symptoms. Yet, after identifying the problem, it became apparent the two girls' fear structures were quite different. While Haley suffered from a social anxiety disorder, Camilla demonstrated perfectionism, a common offshoot of obsessive-compulsive disorder (OCD) and generalized anxiety disorder.

When dealing with OCD, smart talk should not be used. Frequently, children with OCD turn their smart talk into a ritual, which is counterproductive to treatment. Thus, for example, an OCD-prone child, such as Camilla, should not dialogue with Worrybug or Germ Worm. Chapter 10 addresses OCD-specific tools and techniques.

If Your Child Doesn't Like Smart Talk

Do not expect the use of smart talk to completely counter an anxiety reaction. Smart talk is one tool among many that can help you and your child manage her anxiety. Some children benefit a great deal from using smart talk; others may not. Similarly, some children gravitate toward using smart talk, while others don't. Even if your child doesn't especially like using smart talk, she can benefit from the process required to generate smart talk. Therefore, I recommend working through the process, whether or not you child ultimately uses smart talk. However, I *never* force it on a child who doesn't find it useful after several attempts.

Expectations for Smart Talk

It is important to maintain realistic expectations regarding the use of smart talk. Don't expect your child to suddenly respond to reason merely because you have introduced this tool. The next time your child becomes frightened of a dog, you do *not* want to say, "Now, remember, we talked about this, and it's not rational to believe that every dog is going to bite you." Instead, employ all the tools at your disposal.

Begin by asking, "Is that Worrybug? What is your fear thermometer rating? Might you use your smart talk?" The goal is for your child to talk to himself using the smart talk phrase you and he agreed upon. Younger children, especially, benefit from gentle and encouraging reminders from their parents.

SUMMARY: What Did You Learn from This Chapter?

- Anxious children make numerous and frequent thinking errors without realizing it.
- Making thinking errors serves to engender and reinforce anxiety because children believe their erroneous thoughts when their anxiety spikes.
- Common thinking errors children make include catastrophizing, futurizing, overprobabilizing, black-and-white thinking, and mind reading.
- Parents are usually adept at recognizing their child's thinking errors but typically respond in ways

that unintentionally reinforce the anxiety.

- Smart talk offers children and parents a constructive way to respond to and correct thinking errors.
- To use smart talk, identify the thinking error, evaluate the evidence through guided discovery, generate the smart talk, and practice the smart talk.
- Engaging in the process of generating smart talk is useful even if your child ultimately does not use it as a tool.

CHAPTER 8

Develop a Plan for Exposures

If you have followed the steps outlined in the preceding chapters, you are ready to embark on what will be most helpful for your child to conquer her fears: exposures. As I stated in chapter 1, "exposure" refers to gradual, repeated contact with the situations that trigger your child's fears while she resists engaging in avoidance and safety behaviors. You can think of an exposure as an experiment. The goal is for your child to learn that the undesirable outcomes she fears in trigger situations either don't occur or are tolerable if they do.

In this chapter, I will describe the different types of exposures you can use. You will then set up exposure experiments for your child, construct an *exposure ladder* together, and implement it. This phase of treatment builds on what you have done in the preceding chapters.

Types of Exposures

There are three main types of exposures: *in vivo* exposures, imaginal exposures, and exposures to body sensations of anxiety (or interoceptive exposures). You may use one or more of these types with your child, depending on what you find most effective and what is most appropriate for your child's fears.

In Vivo Exposures

In vivo exposures are exposures that are done in real-life situations. When creating in vivo exposures, it is important to select situations that match your child's fear structure. For example, if the downward arrow technique reveals that he specifically fears being sniffed—or worse, licked—by a dog, the exposure needs to include sniffing and licking (likely done by enlisting a familiar dog), rather than just being close to the dog.

I include the use of photographs, videos, and other representational elements in the in vivo exposure category. YouTube videos and Google images are great sources. You will find videos or images for just about any fear your child might have. However, be sure to preview all videos and images for age appropriateness before you use them with your child.

Imaginal Exposures

Imaginal exposures involve asking your child to imagine he is in a specific trigger situation. Imaginal exposure is especially useful when (1) the situation infrequently or never occurs in real life, (2) the fear itself is a thought or image, or (3) he is completely avoiding the situation and his fear thermometer rating is too high to use an in vivo exposure at the outset.

Imaginal exposures are most effective when a child is able to engage all his senses. Thus, you want to encourage him to imagine what he might be seeing, hearing, smelling, tasting, and feeling in an imagined situation. You may need to prompt him to elicit a fully realized imaginal exposure by asking questions:

- "What are the sounds you hear while riding the bus?" (if your child fears vomiting while riding the school bus)
- "How close are you standing to the boy? Is he looking at you?" (if your child fears thoughts about hurting others)
- "What does the room look like? Can you hear the clock ticking?" (if your child is too afraid to physically go to the room)

Some children have a natural facility for imaginal exposures, while others struggle to envision a situation. If your child can engage fully with his imagination, he is likely to have a high fear thermometer response to an imaginal exposure. In this case, imaginal exposures can be therapeutic and play a useful role in recovery. However, if imaginal exposure produces little or no anxious reaction in your child, this type of exposure may not be effective. To be effective, imagining being in a trigger situation needs to produce a fear thermometer rating of at least 1 or 2.

Note that children sometimes get confused by imaginal exposures and think they are being asked to estimate their fear thermometer rating for an in vivo exposure. If this happens, you can clarify by saying, for example, "I understand your fear thermometer rating would be a 10 if you had to actually touch a snake. But what would it be if you just imagined touching one?" If you sense that your child still cannot tell the difference, imaginal exposures are probably not the best method.

Exposures to Body Sensations of Anxiety

Often anxiety is accompanied by a physiological component that can be powerful and dramatic. Many children are frightened by the sensations they have, which include a racing heart, dizziness, nausea, trembling, shortness of breath, hyperventilation, hot flashes, sweating, cold flashes, chest pain, tightness or pressure in the chest, tunnel vision, and tingling. In fact, the sensations themselves and the fear of having them are central to panic disorder. Children with this disorder are on the lookout for these sensations and quickly become fearful when they are evoked.

To expose children to sensations, we use *interoceptive exposures.* This is not as complicated as the term sounds; it is simply a fancy way of saying the exposure involves body sensations. Hyperventilating on purpose or running in place are effective ways to do this because they can bring on sensations that closely mimic those your child fears. The specifics of how to do interoceptive exposures with your child are outlined in the next chapter.

How to Explain Exposures to Your Child

Start by reminding your child that the purpose of doing exposures is to add lots of green candies to his brain, so that when he faces trigger situations, his brain will pull up non-anxious green candies, rather than scary red ones. One way to explain exposures is to compare them to conducting an experiment. This sounds less threatening than "doing an exposure." The idea of an experiment about oneself both perks a child's curiosity and fosters an objective attitude. Saying that he is going to "test something out" reduces anxiety about the prospect of committing to doing something scary for the rest of his life.

Doing Exposures

To plan exposures with your child, you will use the information you have already gathered: the Parent or Child Monitoring Worksheet, your child's trigger situation list, the results of the downward arrow analysis, the Avoidance and Safety Behaviors I Do in Trigger Situations Worksheet, and the Avoidance and Safety Behaviors I Do With My Child Worksheet. Let's walk through each step.

Step 1. Create a Trigger Situation List

Start by creating a list of all the situations that trigger your child's worries. This will be easy because you have the information you need. Go back to your monitoring data and make a list of all the situations that trigger your child's fears. Verify with your child that the triggers and the fear thermometer ratings on this list are currently accurate. Because you and your child have been working at this for a while, some fear ratings may have changed, and you may have discovered trigger situations you missed before. Add any new situations and arrange all of them in hierarchical order, with the highest ratings at the top and the lowest at the bottom.

Here is the trigger situations list created by eleven-year-old Vashti, who suffers from social anxiety, along with her fear thermometer ratings for being in those situations, in hierarchical order.

- Sleepovers with friends I'm not close to (8)

- Making small talk with kids I don't know well (8)
- Asking for something I need or asking a favor (7)
- Inviting a friend I don't know well for a sleepover (6)
- Attending a birthday party with girls I don't know well (5)
- Greeting other kids with eye contact and saying "hi" (4)
- Walking around school between class without a good friend (4)
- Sleepovers at Diana's (3)

Step 2. Select a Trigger Situation and Identify Any Sub-Situations

Although recent research supports doing exposures in random order rather than starting at the lowest fear thermometer rating, motivating a child to do difficult exposures can be a challenge. Therefore, because we want your child to succeed, I recommend you start with the situation that has the lowest rating. If your child feels motivated to start with a situation that has a higher rating (as we discussed in chapter 5), that is fine, too. However, in my experience, most children are more willing to start with less challenging exposures and work their way up the ladder.

A trigger situation is usually best broken down into several subsituations. If your child perceives a task as less overwhelming and more manageable, he is likely to have greater confidence doing it. Confidence boosts motivation, and this makes it more likely he will succeed. Recognizing sub-situations also makes him aware of the nuances inherent in a situation. You can then use this knowledge to design experiments that accurately target his fear structure, which results in more rapid and longer-lasting progress as he climbs his exposure ladders.

Sometimes the situation that triggers a child's lowest fear thermometer rating happens infrequently. The best strategy in that case is to select a situation that has a higher fear thermometer rating but that can occur regularly. You can break that situation down into subsituations and select the one with the lowest fear thermometer rating for your child's first exposure.

The following dialogue between Vashti and her mother shows how to break down a trigger situation and how to use the information you have about avoidance and safety behaviors in this process.

Parent: Let's see what situation we can pick for your first exposure experiment. It should have a low fear thermometer rating. We want you to start with something pretty easy.

Vashti: Sleepovers at Diana's house are a 3. That would be easiest, I guess.

Parent: True. But we also need something that happens regularly. Diana has sleepovers only once a month.

Vashti: (*looking over the worksheet*) But the ones that are rated 4 are too hard. Like greeting kids I don't even know. I don't want to do that.

Parent: Okay, I understand that. Maybe we can pick something that is similar to sleepovers but more part of your daily routine.

Vashti: Well, I could go over to play with Diana more. That would also be a 3.

Parent: That's great thinking, Vashti! Let's consider that for a minute. It's not on the worksheet. Do you do any avoidance or safety behaviors there?

Vashti: Yup. I'd probably go there more if didn't have to do them.

Parent: Tell me more. What makes you uncomfortable when you go over there?

Vashti: For starters, I might see her older brother.

Parent: You mean Alex might be at home, and you would have to say hi?

Vashti: Uh-huh. Even before that, I get a high rating when I knock on the door.

Parent: What about knocking on the door gives you a high rating?

Vashti: I never know who will answer! It could be Alex, and that makes me nervous—like we've talked about.

Parent: You mean the downward arrow results? You're concerned that if you feel nervous, your mind will go blank, you won't be able to say anything, and then Alex will think you're weird and talk about you to other kids?

Vashti: Yup. Lots of times, I text Diana to tell her I'm there so I don't have to knock.

Parent: You've got the idea. And you just identified another safety behavior, didn't you?

Vashti: I never thought of that. It is a safety behavior. Should we add it to the list?

Parent: Yes. So what would your rating be if you didn't do the texting safety behavior and just knocked on the door?

Vashti: I'd say a 4.

Parent: Let's brainstorm and see how many other sub-situations we can come up with. So far we have knocking on the door. What might come next?

Vashti: I usually go into Diana's room with her.

Parent: Okay, that's good. What fear thermometer rating do you have in her room?

Vashti: None. But after a while we usually go into the kitchen for a snack. If no one else is there, that is a 2.

Parent: What happens if someone else is there?

Vashti: When Alex studies in the kitchen, he talks a lot. Plus, sometimes he has a friend with him, which gives me a higher fear rating.

Parent: What is your rating if Alex has a friend?

Vashti: It could be a 7, especially if I don't know the friend.

Parent: That's a good discovery. We can use the information to help us. What do Alex and his friend talk about?

Vashti: Just normal stuff. How club soccer is going, you know.

Parent: It sounds like they just make small talk.

Vashti: I guess so.

Parent: Good job. What fear rating do you have for small talk with Alex?

Vashti: Probably about a 5.

Parent: Which avoidance and safety behaviors might you be tempted to use in these small talk situations?

Vashti: If I hear people in the kitchen, I just tell Diana I'm fine without a snack.

Parent: What kind of avoidance or safety behavior is that?

Vashti: I guess it is making excuses.

Parent: Right you are! Any other behaviors you might have the urge to use if Diana's family or Alex's friends are in the kitchen when you go for a snack?

Vashti: Sometimes I try to avoid eye contact, so they don't want to talk to me. Or I'll read something, like a magazine, so they think I'm busy.

Parent: Very good. I see those on your Avoidance and Safety Behaviors I Do in Trigger Situations Worksheet. If you didn't do these behaviors, what would your rating be for being in the kitchen with Alex and maybe a friend of his?

Vashti: That would be hard. About a 7.

Parent: Good job. What might come next?

Vashti and her mother would continue in this manner until they are satisfied they have identified the sub-situations that comprise a visit to Diana's house, such as greeting Alex in passing in the house, saying something to Diana in front of Alex, and saying goodbye to Alex. Vashti and her mother then make a list of these sub-situations in hierarchical order. Note that some of the sub-situations—especially those having to do with Alex—have higher ratings than the general situation of visiting Diana's house, which is a 3:

- Being in the kitchen with Alex his friends (7)
- Small talk with Alex (5)
- Saying goodbye to Alex (4)
- Saying something to Diana in front of Alex (4)
- Knocking on the door without texting first (4)
- Knocking on the door after texting (3)
- Greeting Alex in passing (3)
- Having a snack with Diana when Alex is not in the kitchen (2)

Step 3. Create an Exposure Ladder

Now that you have identified the situations and sub-situations to be used in exposures, you are ready to create an exposure ladder. The metaphor of a ladder is one children can easily grasp. It's hard to go straight to the most feared situation (the top rung), so a ladder is used to climb up one manageable rung at a time. It's good to have four or five rungs per ladder, but there are no hard-and-fast rules about this. Some situations will require more rungs than others, depending on how complex and challenging they are for your child. However, you should have a sufficient number so no single step is too difficult. At a minimum, I recommend that each time you sit down with your child to plan exposures, you identify at least one your child can start promptly.

Let's look at the conversation Vashti and her mother had when they were designing an exposure ladder for the situation of visiting Diana's house.

Parent: Vashti, let's start with the sub-situations that have the lowest fear thermometer ratings.

Vashti: Let me see. (*She looks at the sub-situation list and the Avoidance and Safety Behaviors I Do in Trigger Situations Worksheet.*) Going into the kitchen with Diana is between a 2 and a 4. The behavior I'd want to do first is just plain avoidance. Usually I stay in Diana's room as much as possible so I don't have to talk to Alex or meet his friends.

Parent: Good job. You'd want to stay in Diana's room, and you also pretend you're busy so Alex or his friends don't talk to you. Let's take these one at a time. What do you think would happen if you didn't stay in Diana's room so much?

Vashti: What do you mean? I can't stay in Diana's room at all?

Parent: Not exactly. But you said you often ask to do things in her room because you have a high fear rating in the kitchen. Remember, we're planning experiments to help you conquer Worrybug so you'll feel more comfortable visiting Diana.

Vashti: Yes, I remember.

Parent: Let's figure out a plan so you can experiment little by little. That way, it won't feel too difficult.

Vashti: Okay.

Parent: You're being a trooper, Vashti. How about if you start by greeting Alex with eye contact? That's between a 2 and a 3 for you, right? That could be the first rung on your ladder. What do you think?

Vashti: I can do it.

Parent: I understand it might be challenging, and I'm so proud of you for being willing to try!

By engaging in a similar discussion, you and your child can choose an initial trigger situation and a rung he feels confident he can manage.

Step 4. Exposure Role-Play Practice

Role-playing is useful to get exposures started. Before I ask a child to do an exposure in real life, we practice it in my office, even if we think it will be relatively easy. If an exposure involves interactions with a same-age or slightly older child, like Vashti's, I will role-play that child. I play up the qualities of that child so the role-playing can be as realistic as possible. You might be surprised: doing this can be fun! Cultivating a sense of humor about the process can also be therapeutic. Encouraging your child to role-play with you ahead of a planned exposure increases the chance of success. Here is how Vashti's mother introduced the idea.

Parent: Why don't we practice a couple of times? Let's go to the front door. I know it seems a little silly, but let's make it as realistic as we can. You stand outside the door, ring the bell, and I'll pretend to be Alex. Remember, it's important you don't do safety or avoidance behaviors—even when we role-play.

Vashti: (*rolling her eyes*) Really, Mom?

Parent: Yes, Vashti, this will help.

Make your role-play as realistic as possible. For example, Vashti's mother will mimic Alex's behavior as closely as she can to duplicate the experience Vashti is likely to have doing her first exposure. In all likelihood, your child will have an anxiety response to the role-play. This is great because it provides an opportunity for exposure and shows you are on the right track. Ask her for a fear thermometer rating if this occurs, and then repeat the role-play until she feels more comfortable with the process. There is no rule regarding how many repetitions you should do. The goal is for her to feel prepared for the real-life exposures.

Step 5. Running the Exposure Experiment

You and your child should soon feel ready to formally run the first experiment. I recommend you pick a specific day and time for each experiment. This greatly increases the likelihood your child will get the job done. If you simply suggest she try to do the experiment when she can, she may procrastinate, delay, and avoid. Set a tone of accountability and back it up with a review of the reward she will earn for doing her exposure in a timely fashion.

Before beginning the experiment, have your child complete the Before Exposure Worksheet. You will find a blank copy in appendix G (http://www. newharbinger.com/39539). The last question is important. It asks your child about her level of confidence in doing the exposure without engaging in avoidance or safety behaviors (high, medium, or low). If she doesn't feel highly confident she can do an exposure, even if her fear thermometer rating suggests otherwise, consider making the exposure easier. If your child struggles to give a confidence rating, try asking her to imagine doing the exposure. Here is how Vashti answered the Before Exposure Worksheet questions:

Vashti's Before Exposure Worksheet

What I plan to do: *Knock on Diana's front door*

What am I most worried will happen? *Alex will answer the door. I will get so nervous that I won't be able to talk. Alex will laugh at me and then tell other kids at school I am weird.*

How will I know if this happens? *I will know if I can't talk. I will hear Alex laugh at me. I won't know right away if he talks about me to other kids, but I'll worry about it, and eventually kids will ignore me or not want to be my friend.*

How strongly do I believe my prediction is correct (0–100%)? *50%*

What will my fear thermometer rating be? *4*

Which safety or avoidance behaviors might I want to do? *Text Diana ahead of time.*

How confident do I feel that I can do the exposure without doing avoidance or safety behaviors? High? Medium? Low? *High*

After the exposure, congratulate, praise, and hug your child. Provide any promised reward. Have her complete the After Exposure Worksheet, which will help her review what she learned from doing the exposure. You will find a blank copy in appendix H (http://www.newharbinger.com/39539). Here's Vashti's worksheet:

Vashti's After Exposure Worksheet

Did what I was most worried about occur? *No*

What did happen? Was I surprised? *When I got to the door, I was really nervous. I waited for a sec and then pushed myself to knock. Alex answered, and he just said, "Hi,*

> *Vashti!" and Diana came running up. I'm pretty sure I said hi back. Alex went back to his computer. He didn't talk much. I was really surprised Alex didn't notice I was nervous. Maybe he was busy worrying about the history paper he was writing.*
>
> **What was my fear thermometer rating?** *It was a 5 right before I knocked, but then it went down quickly to a 2 after Alex answered the door, and Diana came to get me.*
>
> **What did I learn?** *That what I thought would happen didn't at all. I got super worried, but it was fine.*

Of course you want exposures to go well for your child, as Vashti's did. But what if that doesn't happen? For example, your child's fear thermometer rating may rise significantly more than expected or what she feared may occur to some extent. But even if an exposure is challenging, she can still benefit from learning that she can tolerate feeling anxious. So don't consider any experiment a failure. Focus on what your child learned by running the experiment—and keep at it!

Step 6. Climbing More Rungs on the Exposure Ladder

Your goal is to provide many opportunities for your child to practice exposures. Numerous, frequent, and varied experiments provide him the experiences necessary to learn to be less anxious quickly and easily. After one experiment has been completed, go back to your list and start to create one on the next rung.

It is important to incorporate your child's most feared situation in the exposure ladder. As he successfully completes exposures with low ratings, he will learn to be less fearful, and the ratings for the scariest exposures will fall. Thus, your child also learns a key principle: the more exposures he completes, the easier they get. Your child will probably never have to do an exposure that is a 10, because as he masters each rung of the ladder, the next one will be easier. In this manner, his brain is well on its way to learning it need not fear the situation.

Tips and Troubleshooting: Issues with Exposures

As you devise and complete exposures, you and your child are likely to experience some hiccups and roadblocks. To assist in troubleshooting problems that arise, I have included some tips for resolving them.

Keeping Risks Safe and Knowing Your Limits as a Parent

I never ask any child to do something that could expose her to actual jeopardy. For example, it is reasonable to expect a child to risk feeling embarrassed by doing something most children find unobjectionable. Thus, an exposure that requires your child to go into a bakery and ask if they sell doughnuts might be embarrassing, but it is not unreasonable or unsafe. In fact, it would be a good exposure for a child who fears asking questions and appearing stupid or uncool. Conversely, asking your child to order a hundred doughnuts to be delivered to her tree fort would be inappropriate and could cause problems. Similarly, if your child is afraid of heights, a reasonable exposure would be to require her to stand on the viewing deck of a tall building and peer over the edge. It would not be reasonable, of course, to ask her to stand on the railing of that deck, where she could actually fall.

If your child's fears involve content that is frightening to you (e.g., if your child has aggressive obsessions), it may be best to seek the help of an experienced CBT therapist. I discuss this further in chapter 11.

The Feared Consequence Is Not Immediate

Many anxious children have fears with dreaded consequences that are not expected immediately. For example, Marco fears vomiting, and a child in his class came down with the flu. Marco knows it may take several days to contract the flu after being exposed. In this case, Marco and his parent will want to obtain Marco's predictions for what will happen during that waiting period. The parent can use the downward arrow technique to ascertain what Marco fears will happen in those days—will he be so preoccupied that he won't be able to take a quiz in class, do homework, or sleep at night?

My Child Is Completing Exposures but Is Still Very Anxious

Your child may remain anxious because he is still doing safety behaviors, rituals, or avoidance behaviors. The minds of people with anxiety disorders are remarkably adept at inventing new paths of avoidance. Sit down with him and troubleshoot. Ask what thoughts he is having while doing exposures. For example, he may be engaging in reassuring thoughts, such as *I'll be fine* (safety behavior), or in subtle escape thinking, such as

This will be over in five minutes (avoidance behavior). Establish a reward system that encourages him to eliminate these behaviors. Check in with him about reliance on safety or avoidance behaviors, both before and after doing an exposure. If your child expects such check-ins, he will feel more accountable for any such behaviors. Anxiety is sneaky, and you have to be savvier than it is.

He may also be doing safety behaviors after exposures (rather than during them). This also interferes with learning to be less anxious. If you suspect this is the case, ask him. Explain that these behaviors prevent him from conquering his fears. Again, set up rewards to encourage him to abandon them.

All the Exposures Seem Too Challenging.

Don't be deterred if your child tells you that most of the situations you come up with together are a 10 on the fear thermometer. This is likely an avoidance behavior. Your child may fear that even thinking about a situation will cause her mind to worry more about it. Tell her that many anxious people have this fear, but in fact, the opposite will occur. Explain that this fear is another sign of Worrybug.

Children sometimes initially rate exposures higher than they really are, as well as higher than they might after they become familiar with doing exposures. This can be a strategy to avoid the situation—either consciously or unconsciously. If your child has avoided a particular situation for any period of time, her preferred mode will be to continue to avoid. If she is rating all the proposed exposures above a 5, you will need to break them down into smaller, more manageable steps.

Another option is to start with imaginal exposures and transition to other types of exposures when she feels more comfortable. Don't be concerned about experiments being too easy. When she sees that her expectations of bad outcomes were not accurate, she will begin to trust the process and gain confidence in doing exposures.

As mentioned, challenging exposures are not necessarily a cause for concern. Even if an exposure is distressing, by facing a fear rather than avoiding it, your child has an opportunity to learn that she can manage the situation. In addition to feeling worried about feeling anxious, many children with anxiety problems have a low tolerance for distress in general. They are often extremely sensitive to physical comfort, tactile comfort, noise tolerance, disgust, food preferences, unwanted emotional states, and so on. Thus, exposure to distress itself can be therapeutic.

My Child Is Uncooperative

If your child refuses to cooperate in or throws a temper tantrum about the exposures you have planned, it is possible his fears are so severe that professional guidance is warranted. But another explanation is that he is engaging in avoidance behavior. Screaming, crying, complaining, and mean-spirited comments are tactics some children employ to avoid what they don't want or are afraid to do. If acting out helps them avoid performing exposures, they will exhibit more such behaviors.

First, understand that punishment does not motivate children; rewards do. If your child is not cooperating, try offering a reward for not doing the distressing or annoying avoidance behaviors. Second, identify the behaviors (e.g., whining, slamming doors, and name calling) that he does when being uncooperative. If you notice a pattern, talk to him about it.

Parent: John, I've noticed that whenever I remind you to do your experiments, you seem to get really upset. Lately, you've been slamming the door and throwing things, and one time you even said you hated me.

John: Yeah, I don't like doing them.

Parent: I understand they are difficult. I have a strategy that might help you. Let's go over the behaviors you do when you don't want to do an experiment.

[Adopt a calm, business-like attitude; don't express anger or resentment.]

John: Okay.

Parent: Let's make a list of those behaviors.

John: Well, I slammed the door yesterday.

Parent: Good start. What about throwing things?

John: Yes, I've been doing that. I guess saying I hated you is another one.

[You can write down a list of these behaviors for reference.]
Parent: So far we have slamming the door, throwing things, and name calling. Can you think of anything else?

John: What about when I scream to myself?

Parent: Great. Now we have slamming the door, throwing things, name calling, and screaming. How hard it would be, on a scale of 1 to 10, for you to resist the urge to do any of these things during the first two minutes of your experiment?

John: If I really think about, two minutes would be easy. A 0.

Parent: What about if you resisted for five minutes? How difficult would that be?

John: About a 4.

Parent: Would you be willing to start with two minutes of resisting those behaviors if we set up a reward and I remind you?

John: What would the reward be?

Parent: How about five minutes of video game time on Saturday?

John: Would I get more time if I don't do the behaviors for five minutes?

Parent: Absolutely.

John: Can I add up the time?

Parent: Sure you can. This strategy is effective for behavioral problems whether or not your child suffers from anxiety responses.

The Exposures Are Too Boring

I find that imaginal exposures, especially, can get tedious for children. Some children are great at using their imagination to make things seem real, but others are not. If your child can't elicit a fear thermometer rating for an imaginal exposure or can't make it seem real, switch to another type of exposure. Or your child could try saying imaginal exposures aloud so they feel more real.

That being said, complaints of boredom can be avoidance strategies. If you suspect your child is avoiding an exposure, sit down with her and talk about it in a neutral and factual manner to determine if this is the case. If it is, don't become annoyed or frustrated.

Collaborate with her to forge more manageable steps, such as breaking down situations into sub-situations, and check your own participation in safety or avoidance behaviors.

Another reason your child can be bored by an exposure is that she has learned that nothing terrible happens when doing it. In other words, she has conquered that fear. This, after all, is your goal. Ask if her fears related to the exposure are reduced in real life, as well. If so, she can climb up to the next rung on the exposure ladder.

SUMMARY: What Did You Learn from This Chapter?

- Types of exposures include in vivo, imaginal, and exposure to body sensations.
- Children can understand exposures as experiments in which they can test out whether what they expect to happen in a trigger situation actually occurs.
- Numerous, frequent, and varied experiments provide your child the

experiences necessary to learn to be less anxious quickly and easily.

- The steps to follow when planning exposures include creating a trigger situation list, selecting a situation and identifying possible sub-situations, creating an exposure ladder, role-playing, doing the first exposure, and climbing more rungs.
- A child should never be put in harm's way during an exposure.
- A child who is still anxious despite doing exposures may be engaging in avoidance or safety behaviors during or after exposures.
- If your child finds an exposure too challenging, start with an easier one.
- If your child says an exposure is boring, he may be using avoidance behaviors, or he may have already conquered that fear.

CHAPTER 9

Find Exposures That Work

The specific exposures you plan with your child need to directly relate to his fear structure. In this chapter, you will find examples of different types of exposures for different kinds of fears and anxieties—separation anxiety, social anxiety, fear of animals and bugs, environmental fears, eating worries, health worries, blood and injection worries, and panic attacks and body sensation fears. Some examples will be just right for your child, while others may not be an exact fit, and you will have to apply the knowledge you've gleaned thus far and extrapolate.

First review the types of fears described to identify which match your child's. If more than one type is applicable, select the one that fits best. Then pick a quiet time to sit down with your child and ask him to give a fear thermometer rating for each trigger situation for which I have suggested an exposure. A high rating indicates you are on the right track. If he says he would want to use his avoidance or safety behaviors in a particular situation, you are also likely on the right track. In this case (as you did when using the downward arrow technique), ask what he predicts will happen if he does not engage in those behaviors in that situation.

Remember to break trigger situations down into sub-situations. Invite your child to actively participate in planning exposures for those situations. Ask him for ideas. After all, he knows best which situations are the biggest triggers. Children often enjoy lending their expertise and participating in this way. The more your child participates, the more he owns the process. Use his input to help you understand the intricacies of his fears and to construct optimally effective experiments.

The exposures your child does should elicit a response. You may be surprised by his reactions. Some exposures you expect to be effective will fail to produce a fear thermometer rating. Ones you expect to be innocuous may elicit a high rating and thus be of great therapeutic value. For this reason, I have provided a wide range of exposure ideas as a starting point for your child's personal plan. And don't hesitate to ask your child questions you think may elicit anxiety. Remember that even when your child talks about what he is afraid of, he will likely experience a fear thermometer surge of some sort. This is a good thing! It tells you that you are on the right track and that your child is already benefitting from the therapeutic effects of exposure.

Separation Anxiety

Separation anxiety is common, especially among younger children. Children worry about losing the comforting presence of a parent when they are separated. They may also fear that harm will come to their parents or loved ones, such that they might not ever return. Extreme homesickness is another form of separation anxiety.

The following exposures can be effective for separation anxiety.

- Spend five (or more) minutes in a room where you are separated from your parent, without knowing exactly where your parent is in the house.
- Spend time in the backyard, without knowing where your parent is in the house.
- Allow your parents to leave the house for five (or more) minutes, without knowing where they are going.
- Allow your parents to go out for an hour (while you stay with a sitter), without knowing where they are going.
- Allow your parents to go out for more than an hour (while you stay with a sitter) without knowing where they are going.
- Allow your parents to go on an overnight (while you stay with a sitter) without knowing where they are going.
- Allow your parents to go away for a weekend while you stay with a sitter) without knowing where they are going.

Six-year-old Lucinda has experienced anxiety upon separation from her parents, especially her mother, since preschool. In preschool, she cried harder and longer than any other child at drop-off times. Each year, she experienced the same level of distress, which persisted for well over a month into each year. Every Sunday, Lucinda became anxious about the upcoming Monday morning separation. Her mother could not leave her with a sitter, even for a short time. Lucinda was like her mother's shadow when at home: she needed to be in the same room as her mother, and if not, she would call out to her mother so she could know her location.

Lucinda and her parents decided her first exposure would be to spend five minutes in a room alone, without knowing where her parents were in the house. Here you can see how Lucinda completed her exposure worksheet with her *parents before running their first experiment.*

Lucinda's Before Exposure Worksheet

What I plan to do: *I will go into the den and stay by myself for 5 minutes while my parents are somewhere else in the house. I won't know where they are, and they will be super quiet so I don't figure it out.*

What am I most worried will happen? *They won't come back; I won't ever see them again.*

How will I know if this happens? *Well, they will just be gone, and I'll wait and wait and wait, and they won't come back.*

How strongly do I believe my prediction is correct (0–100%)? *For 5 minutes, it would be hard for them to disappear. Maybe only 20%?*

What will my fear thermometer rating be? *5*

Which safety or avoidance behaviors might I want to do? *I will want to call out to my parents and have them answer to tell me* *where they are. I will want to run and find them.*

How confident do I feel that I can do the exposure without doing avoidance or safety behaviors? High? Medium? Low? *I can do it. It's just 5 minutes. High*

Social Anxiety

Children with social anxiety fear being judged negatively by others or may be uncomfortable being the center of attention. The following exposures can be effective for social anxiety.

- Make eye contact with someone who triggers a high fear rating.
- Say hi while making eye contact with someone who triggers a high fear rating.
- Make eye contact with a kid at school who is a casual acquaintance.
- Say hi while making eye contact with a child at school who is a casual acquaintance.
- Ask a store clerk a simple question.

- Ask a store clerk a detailed question.
- Make a special request to a store clerk, such as "Do you have brownies?" when you do not see them available.
- Make phone calls and ask a simple question. [Compile a list of twenty or more businesses (e.g., a pizza parlor, dry cleaner, pet store) in your area and ask your child to call each and ask one question.]
- Call a relative to ask a question.
- Call a friend and invite him or her to an event or outing.
- Place your own order in a restaurant.
- Make a special request in a restaurant.
- Ask a silly question, such as "Do you sell doughnuts?" in a doughnut shop. [Useful for worries about being embarrassed.]
- Ask a stranger for directions (with adult supervision, of course).
- Take a taxi with a parent and tell the driver your destination.
- Answer the phone at home without knowing who is calling.

- Raise your hand in class to ask a question.
- Be the center of attention by doing something noticeable in public (e.g., sing, do a cartwheel, laugh loudly, wear something flashy, drop your books on the ground).
- Return an item to a store. [Good for anxiety about inconveniencing others.]
- Pretend you forgot your money when you get to the cash register. [Good for anxiety about inconveniencing others.]
- Be extra slow at doing something. [Good for anxiety about inconveniencing others.]
- Mumble or stumble on your words a little on purpose.
- Pause too long between two words.
- Tremble or shake a little on purpose.

Twelve-year-old Juan is friendly and popular. He plays soccer and gets straight As. However, he experiences a lot of anxiety when he is the center of attention—when he is called on in class, when his soccer coach instructs him in front of the team, and when he is late to class. He is creative about avoiding these situations. He speaks with his teachers outside class, so they will be less likely to call on him (a safety behavior). He makes excuses for not trying out for major roles in the school play, even though his friends and drama teacher tell him he'd be great. Parents are often perplexed when a child (like Juan) does not show the obvious signs of social anxiety, such as shyness and discomfort, because they have no reason to think he has difficulty engaging in social activities. However, the same kinds of exposures will work. Juan could do the experiment of raising his hand in class, or he could do an experiment that makes him the center of attention in a social situation.

Juan decided to do the experiment of dropping his books at school as a start, even though he gave it a fear thermometer rating of 6, because it gets to the heart of his worry about being the *center of attention. You can see how he completed his Before Exposure Worksheet.*

Juan's Before Exposure Worksheet

What I plan to do: *Drop a stack of my books in the hallway between classes.*

What am I most worried will happen? *Everyone will stop and look at me. They will all stare. I will feel nervous and turn red with embarrassment. Kids will laugh at me.*

How will I know if this happens? *I will see them staring at me and hear them laughing.*

How strongly do I believe my prediction is correct (0–100%)? *60%*

What will my fear thermometer rating be? *6*

Which avoidance or safety behaviors might I want to do? *Pick up my books as fast as I can.*

How confident do I feel that I can do the exposure without doing

avoidance or safety behaviors?
High? Medium? Low? *High*

Fears of Animals or Bugs

Fears of animals or bugs are quite common. The following exposures can be effective for these fears.

- Look at pictures of a feared animal or insect in a book or on the Internet.
- View YouTube videos of feared creatures in action. [Particularly in situations similar to those your child fears, such as off-leash dogs or a cat licking someone.]
- Visit an animal shelter and view live animals from outside the pen.
- Visit a familiar animal that is not in a pen or cage, while standing at a specified distance.
- Stand at a specified distance from a leashed or otherwise controlled creature.
- Stand at a specified distance from an unleashed, free-roaming known creature.

- Touch a known animal that is leashed or otherwise controlled.
- Touch a known animal that is unleashed or free roaming.
- Pet an animal that is leashed or otherwise controlled.
- Pet an animal that is unleashed or free roaming.
- Visit an off-leash dog park.
- Allow a dog to lick you.
- Feed a dog a treat.
- Purchase ladybugs at a nursery to view.
- Purchase ladybugs and allow them to crawl on your body (e.g., arm, hair).
- Imagine a dog running at you.
- Imagine petting a dog.
- Imagine a dog licking you.

From the downward arrow technique results for eight-year-old Henry, he and his parents knew that he fears an off-leash dog will bite him. One first experiment Henry could do would be to stand for five minutes on the sidelines of his sister's soccer game while an off-leash dog is present. Another experiment would be to stand quietly for five minutes when Duke (a neighbor's dog that often comes over and wants Henry to throw a ball for him) approaches him. Henry chose to go to his sister's soccer game because that was easier than the experiment with Duke. He gave standing at the sidelines while off-leash dogs were present a rating of 4. This is how Henry filled out the worksheet before doing this experiment.

Henry's Before Exposure Worksheet

What I plan to do: *Stand on the sideline at Melissa's soccer game when off-leash dogs are close by.*

What am I most worried will happen? *A dog will come up to me and bite me or jump up on me.*

How will I know if this happens? *It will be obvious because I'll have a dog bite or people will see a dog jump up on me.*

How strongly do I believe my prediction is correct (0–100%)? *20%*

What will my fear thermometer rating be? *4*

Which avoidance or safety behaviors might I want to do? *Stand away from dogs. Stand right next to my mom or dad. Watch for off-leash dogs.*

How confident do I feel that I can do the exposure without doing avoidance or safety behaviors? High? Medium? Low? *High*

Environmental Fears

Environmental fears include heights, crowds, elevators, airplanes, natural disasters (e.g., fires, storms), wind, thunder, loud noises, uncomfortable clothing, and other similar concerns. The following exposures can be used to target environmental fears.

- Look at photos of fires, storms, tornados, or other natural disasters.
- Read newspaper articles about fires, storms, fires, or other natural disasters.

- Watch news broadcasts of natural disasters and record for repeated viewing.
- Watch YouTube coverage of natural disasters.
- Listen to audio of thunder, lightning, high wind, or airplane flight noises.
- Watch movies of natural disasters that show the damage.
- Ride the elevator in a tall building.
- Watch YouTube coverage of an airplane flight (not involving accidents).
- Pack your suitcase for an airplane trip.
- Imagine flying on an airplane, including takeoff and landing.
- Listen to the audio of a flight: in-cabin sounds, flight announcements.
- Go to crowded places, with varying levels of noise and crowd density.
- Watch live concert coverage.
- Wear clothing items that have an itchy tag, a seam in socks, or other slightly uncomfortable qualities.
- Imagine a fire breaking out near you.

- Imagine a tornado approaching your home.

Beth is an eleven-year-old who fears crowded places and loud noise. She refuses to go to movies, athletic events, and concerts. Her brother Chad made the high school football team and wants her to watch him play. However, she is afraid she will faint if she is in the large and noisy crowd. In the event of a terror attack, she fears she would be trapped and unable to get out.

Beth could do an experiment of watching a football practice instead of going to a game. She could also watch a video of a game and imagine she is there in person. Another experiment she could do would be to imagine a terror attack happening. She decided to watch a video of the homecoming game her brother played in. She gave this experiment a fear thermometer rating of 4. She chose this because it would be easier than going to a game or even to a practice. Here is her Before Exposure Worksheet

Beth's Before Exposure Worksheet

What I plan to do: *Watch a video of the homecoming game with the volume turned up. Imagine I'm there, hearing the loudness and being in the crowd.*

What am I most worried will happen? *I will feel really nervous. I will feel more scared to be at the next game.*

How will I know if this happens? *I will have a high fear thermometer rating. I won't go to the next home game, even though it won't be super crowded.*

How strongly do I believe my prediction is correct (0–100%)? *20%*

What will my fear thermometer rating be? *4*

Which avoidance or safety behaviors might I want to do? *I might want to turn down the volume or remind myself I'm not really there. Not go to the next game.*

**How confident do I feel that I can do the exposure without doing

avoidance or safety behaviors?
High? Medium? Low? *High*

Eating Worries

Children can develop worries about eating food. The fears addressed here do not include eating disorders (e.g., anorexia nervosa, binge-eating disorders, and bulimia), which arise from body image worries and fears of being fat. Children can fear choking on certain foods, swallowing pills, and having undesirable reactions to foods (e.g., feeling overly full or excessively hungry, getting food poisoning, feeling anxious after eating, or having an allergic reaction). They can also fear trying new or different foods and eating foods with certain textures, colors, or smells. Eating worries can also be a sign of health-related or body-focused obsessions and compulsions.

The following exposure ideas can be used to target eating worries.

- Imagine eating a potato chip, chunk of meat, or a hard or dense food.

- Watch a sibling or friend eat the feared food.
- Eat a small piece of the feared food.
- Eat a medium-sized piece of the feared food.
- Smell food with an objectionable odor.
- Eat a food with an undesirable texture (e.g., squishy, slimy, drippy).
- Eat a food with an objectionable color.
- Swallow a very small candy (have your parents cut one up, if necessary).
- Swallow an empty gel capsule.
- Eat an unfamiliar food.
- Go to an unfamiliar restaurant.
- Order an unfamiliar food at a restaurant.
- Combine two to three types of food in one mouthful.
- Drink a mystery smoothie.
- Eat a hamburger or other meat that is pink on the inside.
- Try a different brand of a preferred food.

Seven-year-old Lonnie fears swallowing pills and eating certain foods. He thinks he might choke and die. One experiment Lonnie could do is to swallow a small soft or even a hard candy while refraining from engaging in any safety behaviors, such as aborted attempts or swallowing more water than necessary. Lonnie and his father would arrange several small candies on a plate and sort them by size. When Lonnie has successfully swallowed the smallest size, he can experiment with a larger size.

Lonnie decided to begin with the exposure of swallowing a very small candy with a single sip of water. He gave this experiment a fear thermometer rating of 5. Here is the worksheet he filled out before doing this experiment.

Lonnie's Before Exposure Worksheet

What I plan to do: *Swallow a very small hard candy with only one sip of water.*

What am I most worried will happen? *It will get caught in my throat, and I will choke and maybe die.*

How will I know if this happens? *I will choke and gag. I will stop breathing.*

How strongly do I believe my prediction is correct (0–100%)? *20%*

What will my fear thermometer rating be? *5*

Which avoidance or safety behaviors might I want to do? *Take extra sips of water. Or just not swallow it.*

How confident do I feel that I can do the exposure without doing avoidance or safety behaviors? High? Medium? Low? *Medium. It will be hard for me to not drink extra water.*

Health Worries

Common health worries include contracting diseases, such as cancer, tuberculosis, Ebola, measles, or meningitis. Many children also fear that a bump, headache, or rash is a sign of cancer or another serious condition. Hypochondriasis (i.e., a condition characterized by frequent and extreme concern about one's health) falls into this category. Safety behaviors children with health-related worries use include searching the Internet, avoiding contact with people who might be ill, seeking lots of reassurance, and requesting doctors' office visits. Of course, all physical symptoms must be cleared by a physician so you can be certain no actual illness exists.

The following exposure ideas can be used to target health worries.

- Write a scary word (e.g., cancer, death) and view it repeatedly.
- Say the scary disease word aloud repeatedly.
- Read about the feared disease on the Internet or in medical journals.
- Imagine you have a disease.

- Visit a hospital.
- Watch a video on YouTube of someone vomiting.
- Listen to vomiting sounds (the Internet abounds with such opportunities).
- Pretend to vomit in a toilet with water, then add bits of food and include vomiting sounds.
- Make and view fake vomit (use your imagination: oatmeal, orange juice, yogurt, chunks of tomato, etc.).
- Slop fake vomit on the floor.
- Slop fake vomit on the floor while making vomiting noises.

Nine-year-old Pablo fears he will contract various medical conditions, including a brain tumor, tuberculosis, hepatitis, head lice, and the flu. He continually tells his parents about symptoms he thinks he has and seeks their reassurance that he is okay. His worrying is so severe that it affects his sleep and his schoolwork.

Pablo could to an experiment that involves writing down the word for or a phrase relating to one of the conditions he fears getting. He could also experiment with speaking that word or phrase aloud. He decides to start with the exposure of writing down a phrase about getting a brain tumor. He gave this experiment a fear thermometer rating of 3 to 4. This is the Exposure Worksheet he filled out before doing this experiment.

Pablo's Before Exposure Worksheet

What I plan to do: *Write the phrase "I will get a brain tumor soon."*

What am I most worried will happen? *I will worry more. I won't be able to think of anything else. I won't be able to pay attention in class, do my homework, sleep well, or study for the vocabulary test on Friday.*

How will I know if this happens? *I will get a bad grade on the vocabulary test. I will worry all through class. I will be very tired.*

How strongly do I believe my prediction is correct (0–100%)? *30% I probably won't think about it* *all the time and eventually I will fall asleep.*

What will my fear thermometer rating be? *3–4*

Which avoidance or safety behaviors might I want to do? *I will want to ask my mom if she thinks I'm really going to get a brain tumor because I'm writing about it. I will want to write down that I won't get a tumor.*

How confident do I feel that I can do the exposure without doing avoidance or safety behaviors? High? Medium? Low? *High*

Blood and Injection Fears

Some children have extreme fears of injections, blood draws, and other dental and medical procedures. The following exposure ideas can be used to target these kinds of fears.

- View YouTube videos of blood draws.
- View photos of bloody wounds.
- Handle a bloody object, such as red meat.

- Place fake blood on yourself or others.
- Have your parent prick his or her own finger and show you the blood.
- Have your parent prick his or her own finger, then touch your parent's blood.
- View videos of injections.
- Observe someone getting an injection.
- Have your parent obtain a syringe, alcohol swab, and tourniquet and practice giving you a fake shot (instead of a needle, use a paper clip or something slightly sharp to give the impression of a shot).
- Poke your skin slightly to elicit a low level of pain.
- View photos of medical procedures.
- View videos of medical procedures.
- Visit a medical office and room where procedures occur (e.g., examining table, instruments).
- Read about the possible risks and side effects of various medical procedures.

Ten-year-old Casey has intense fears about going to the doctor, especially if she thinks she may have to get any shots. She recently missed getting a tetanus booster because she feared the pain and possibility of seeing her own blood. Her mother set up another appointment for the shot, as well as for a flu shot. Casey could do an experiment that involves watching a video of a blood draw or an injection or accompany a friend who is getting a vaccine. Or her parents could obtain a syringe for her to handle and practice giving a fake shot.

Casey decided to start by focusing on her fear of blood before dealing with her fear of injections. She agreed to watch a video of a blood draw ten times. She gives this experiment a fear thermometer rating of 4. Here is the worksheet she filled out before doing this experiment.

Casey's Before Exposure Worksheet

What I plan to do: *Watch a video of a blood draw 10 times.*

What am I most worried will happen? *I will feel anxious and even more scared of the upcoming vaccine I have to get.*

How will I know if this happens? *I will have a high fear thermometer rating. I will think about getting the shot constantly. As a result, I will get Bs and not the As I want.*

How strongly do I believe my prediction is correct (0–100%)? *30%*

What will my fear thermometer rating be? *4*

Which avoidance or safety behaviors might I want to do? *I think I can just watch it. But I might want to talk to my mom about postponing my doctor's appointment or seeing if I can skip the shot.*

How confident do I feel that I can do the exposure without doing avoidance or safety behaviors? High? Medium? Low? *High*

Panic Attacks and Body Sensation Fears

Interoceptive exposures involve exposure to body sensations and can be done in a number of ways. Hyperventilating on purpose is the best way to evoke most of the physical sensations associated with anxiety and is what I most commonly use with patients in my practice.

EXERCISE: Hyperventilation. To hyperventilate for exposures, your child should breathe forcefully in and out at a rapid rate for a predetermined period of time. Usually this requires a very vigorous effort, so it is helpful to have a glass of water handy for any throat dryness. A stopwatch or smartphone timer is also necessary. You can use the following steps when teaching your child to hyperventilate.

1. Demonstrate to your child how to take rapid, full breaths in and out.
2. Ask if she is willing to try five to ten breaths to see what it's like.

[If she refuses even five breaths, consider jumping jacks, or other methods suggested here.]

3. Proceed with the five to ten breaths.

4. Ask her to rate how scary the sensations were using the fear thermometer.

5. Ask her how similar the sensation engendered by hyperventilation is to what she experiences when feeling panicked. Have her reply using a scale of 1 to 10, where 1 means the manufactured sensation and feeling of panic are very different and 10 means they are the same. Ideally, the sensations engendered are very similar to those she experiences when feeling panicky.

6. Agree on a length of time to do this exercise. I recommend twenty seconds, but if your child is only willing to do a shorter time, go with that.

7. Have her complete a Before Exposure Worksheet.

8. Do the experiment for twenty seconds.

9.   Have her complete an After Exposure Worksheet.

When she is comfortable with twenty seconds, you can increase the time to thirty seconds, and later to one minute. Most children acclimate physically to this type of exposure quickly. The first few tries usually result in the highest level of dizziness and other sensations, and then the exposure loses its impact after several repetitions. When this occurs, take a break from these exposures. However, you can practice them from time to time even after your child has conquered them.

If you don't feel comfortable asking your child to hyperventilate on purpose, you can achieve interoceptive exposure to the kinds of sensations he fears through one of the following exposures.

- Run in place until breathing hard to create a rapid heart rate.
- Spin in a swivel chair to evoke dizziness.
- Breathe through a thin straw to evoke a sense of restricted air.

- Perform a rapid series of jumping jacks.
- Swallow several times in a row, as quickly as you can [for fears of throat tightness].
- Artificially restrict airflow through the nose with your fingers while breathing through your nose, with your mouth closed.
- Do vigorous exercise in the heat (within reason, of course).
- Use a space heater and coats and scarves to elicit the sensations of overheating.

Ten-year old-Tina witnessed a girl her age having an asthma attack at a soccer game. Since then, she panics in any situation she associates with breathing hard. She refuses to participate in soccer practice, participate in physical education classes, or exert herself physically to the point of breathing hard. Tina has no history of asthma or breathing difficulties. Doing an experiment with hyperventilation could be a good way to help her discover that she can tolerate the breathlessness and panic that she fears.

Tina decided to start with the exposure of hyperventilating for twenty seconds. She gave this experiment a fear thermometer rating of 4. Here is the worksheet she filled out before doing this experiment.

Tina's Before Exposure Worksheet

What I plan to do: *Do a hyperventilation exercise for 20 seconds.*

What am I most worried will happen? *I will feel super dizzy, I might have an asthma attack or pass out.*

How will I know if this happens? *I can tell you that I'm dizzy. I will know if I pass out. I will start to wheeze and not be able to breathe.*

How strongly do I believe my prediction is correct (0–100%)? *100% that I'll get dizzy. 20% that I'll pass out. 10% that I'll have an asthma attack.*

> **What will my fear thermometer rating be?** *4*
>
> **Which avoidance or safety behaviors might I want to do?** *I will want to lie down until I don't feel dizzy.*
>
> **How confident do I feel that I can do the exposure without doing avoidance or safety behaviors? High? Medium? Low?** *I can do it. High confidence.*

SUMMARY: What Did You Learn from This Chapter?

- Exposures need to directly relate to your child's fear structure.
- Exposure ideas for children with separation anxiety include spending five minutes in a separate room in the same house as the parent and allowing parents to leave the house without having knowledge of their location.
- Exposure ideas for children who fear being judged negatively by others include asking questions or

interacting with strangers and speaking in class.

- Exposure ideas for children who fear animals or bugs include looking at photos or videos, being in close proximity, and touching them.
- Exposure ideas for children with environmental fears include looking at photos or videos of disasters and going to a crowded place.
- Exposure ideas for children with eating worries include smelling or eating an unfamiliar or undesirable food.
- Exposure ideas for children with health worries include writing or speaking a scary disease word, making fake vomit, and visiting a hospital.
- Exposure ideas for children with blood or injection fears include viewing blood, an injection, or a medical procedure.
- Hyperventilation can be used for exposures to evoke the physical sensation associated with anxiety.

CHAPTER 10

Manage Obsessive-Compulsive Disorder

Obsessive-compulsive disorder (OCD) is a type of anxiety disorder that is treated a little differently than other anxiety disorders, so I am giving it special attention. According to the American Academy of Child and Adolescent Psychiatry (2013), one in two hundred children and adolescents suffers from it. OCD can manifest at any time between the preschool years and adulthood, but approximately one-third of adults with OCD first experienced symptoms as children. These statistics likely underestimate how many people have OCD, because it is so often misdiagnosed.

OCD involves the presence of both obsessions and compulsion. *Obsessions* engender fear, and *compulsions* (rituals) are then used to quell fear and the accompanying distress. In the same manner, compulsions serve a purpose similar to that of safety behaviors. Although the range of obsessions is far greater than can be addressed here, OCD experts have established categories for the types of obsessions and compulsions that people of all ages, genders, races, and socioeconomic statuses experience. Numerous scholarly books specifically address OCD in children. My goal is to give you a working knowledge of this disorder to help you identify the obsessions and rituals your child is engaging in and to give you guidelines to help him manage this problem.

Obsessions

Obsessions are unwanted recurrent and consistent thoughts, worries, images, urges, or impulses that cause distress and fear. The sufferer's brain overvalues the particular disturbing thought and becomes mired in it. *Overvaluing* means the sufferer believes that because he had that thought, it must be important or true.

Of course, people without OCD—of all ages—can experience distressing thoughts, images, and impulses about many things. This is a normal phenomenon that has been studied. These thoughts can be extreme, bizarre, violent, or sexually disturbing, but the individuals are able to dismiss them. When people without OCD have such a thought, they likely simply think, *Well, that was weird.* They realize that just because the thought occurred doesn't mean they should take it seriously. Most would dismiss such a thought as they would a piece of junk mail. A child suffering from OCD, on the other hand, gets stuck on the thought and experiences a great deal of distress. This leads her to feel she must do a ritual of some kind (a compulsion) to alleviate the fear, make the disturbing thought go away, or be certain the feared consequences the obsession has introduced will not occur.

OCD is an anxiety disorder, but not all anxious children have OCD. The main difference between OCD and other anxiety disorders is that children with OCD perform rituals (mentally or behaviorally) that are repetitive and to which they rigidly adhere. For example, a child with generalized anxiety disorder worries excessively about things that tend to relate to real-life concerns (grades, performance in sports, or global warming), but he won't perform rituals in response. A child with OCD suffering from perfectionistic obsessions will perform rituals, such as insisting on using a certain color pen for particular subjects or repeatedly checking binders, checking work for errors, or checking the Internet for signs of increased global warming.

Obsessions can sometimes involve *excessive guilt* or *excessive responsibility* about particular situations. By *excessive,* I mean more than is typical for the average child. We see these hallmarks of OCD in children with various types of obsessions and sometimes simply in a pure form. For example, a child may refuse a gift to quell the obsession that she has more than others or that others suffer more than she does, while a child with an average sense of guilt would likely feel lucky and accept the gift. Similarly, a child with excessive guilt might become extremely worried if he accidentally damaged something slightly, while a child with reasonable guilt would feel sorry but would accept that it was an honest error and move on.

TABLE 8. Common Obsessions

Obsession	Qualities
Contamination	Concerns about germs, dirt, items perceived as "yucky" or "dirty," chemicals, environmental pollutants (asbestos, pesticides, lead), spoiled food, soap, dead animals, garbage, sticky substances, radioactivity, broken glass, bodily excretions, and magical types of contaminants (certain words, thoughts, names, images, colors)
Intrusive images and thoughts	Graphic mental images about things such as death, murder, and violence
Scrupulosity	Fear of offending God or not believing in God (when that is important to the person); fear of cheating, stealing, or doing other things the person considers immoral
Aggressive	Fear of hurting others or oneself or of harm befalling oneself
Perfectionist	Doubts about remembering, understanding, or knowing things thoroughly; concerns about making errors or omissions, or losing things
Health	Concerns about contracting an illness, disease, or disability not related to contamination
Superstitious or magical	Beliefs that certain numbers, colors, and so on have an important impact
Ordering and arranging	Need to arrange items according to specific spatial patterns or levels of neatness
Thought-action fusion	Belief that having a thought will result in doing something undesirable or forbidden

Obsessions are more varied than educated laypeople or even many mental health professionals are trained to recognize. The obsessions I see most commonly in my practice are listed in table 8, though the table doesn't list all the obsessions children experience.

Compulsions

Compulsions are also known as "rituals"; the terms are interchangeable. Compulsions are repetitive behaviors or thoughts a person engages in to suppress or neutralize obsessions, prevent the feared consequences, and reduce distress. Compulsions take many forms and are performed consciously. A person with OCD decides to engage in a compulsion because it provides temporary relief or assurance the feared consequence will not ensue. Over time, rituals become habits that sufferers have great difficulty resisting when facing a trigger situation. Your child may feel he must do a ritual (in a very particular manner) to make it through that situation. As with avoidance and safety behaviors, rituals provide temporary relief but reinforce obsessions and prevent him from conquering OCD. Keep in mind that obsessions may be less obvious to you than the rituals that accompany them (see table 9). Indeed, a good way to identify an obsession is to watch for the corresponding rituals.

Obsessions and compulsions often have magical qualities that won't make logical sense to you. For example, some children believe that particular numbers carry significance (either good or bad), and they do rituals that include those numbers or are repeated a particular number of times. Compulsions can also be enacted according to specific rules unique to and developed by the sufferer. Your child may fear deviating from the prescribed way of doing a ritual and therefore feel the need to repeat it until it is "done right." Compulsions can also be done mentally, which can make them more challenging to spot.

TABLE 9. Common Types of Rituals

Ritual	Behaviors
Avoidance	Avoiding situations or stimuli that trigger an obsession
Analyzing	Trying to determine why a particular thought, image, or impulse exists
Washing	Handwashing, showering, brushing and flossing teeth, laundering
Creating "clean" rooms	Trying to maintain a safe, clean room or area; disallowing contaminated people or items in that space
Cleaning	Cleaning household or personal items; taking measures to remove contact with contaminants
Throwing items away	Discarding articles to eliminate contamination
Ordering and arranging	Straightening, ordering, and arranging according to particular standards
Symmetry	Evening up behaviors, often involving touching and rearranging
Checking	Checking locks, doors, school books, or homework; checking that no harm has come to someone; checking that nothing terrible did or will happen (newspapers, weather forecasts); checking for mistakes while reading, writing, or making choices
Touching and tapping	Repeated touching, often related to symmetry worries and magical thinking obsessions

Counting, number significance	Counting things; ascribing magical significance to certain numbers (*I'll have a good day if I brush my teeth thirty strokes but have a terrible day if I don't do the correct number of strokes*)
Repeating	Rereading, erasing, rewriting, or needing to repeat routine activities (turning a light switch on and off, going in and out a door, walking up and down a step)
Reassurance seeking	Asking questions or making repeated requests for information
Praying	Praying to neutralize a "bad" or sacrilegious thought
Grooming	Arranging hair in a particular manner
Mental checking	Mentally reviewing a situation
"Just so" or "just right" rituals	Repeating a movement, behavior, thought, or body position until it feels "right"
Confessing	Feeling the need to tell someone about a feared transgression (having a "bad" thought, swearing, being mean to someone, or lying)
Excessive visits to doctor	Repeated trips to physician or emergency room

Identifying OCD in Your Child

More than one type of obsession is usually present, and children and adults alike can do a good job of hiding rituals—especially those performed mentally. Even though you are not a professional, as you learn more about OCD, you'll be better able to recognize and understand your child's obsessions and rituals. To start, answer the questions in the following exercise, which lists behaviors commonly observed in children with OCD.

EXERCISE: Assessing Your Child's OCD.

Does your child *excessively* or *repeatedly*...

- worry about contact with dirt, germs, chemicals, bodily fluids (urine, sweat, feces, saliva), or other substances believed to be harmful?
- wash, bathe, use hand sanitizers, or engage in behaviors (using sleeves, towels) to prevent contact with contaminants?
- worry about being harmed or harming others, either on purpose or accidentally?
- take measures to avoid activities (sports, handling knives and scissors) that could possibly lead to any physical harm to self or others?

- check to be sure no harm has occurred by visually checking and or asking, "Are you okay?"
- worry about contracting diseases or ailments?
- seek reassurance, request visits to the physician, or research illnesses on the Internet?
- do things in a symmetrical fashion, and thus engage in behaviors to even things out (touching, arranging)?
- do things in a manner that feels "just right" (moving body parts, arranging items, saying things, doing routine behaviors)?
- order and arrange items in a precise fashion and feel distressed when such order is disrupted?
- feel the need to complete certain behaviors (homework, art, reading book pages or chapters) and become distressed when interrupted?
- feel the need to express a thought or ask a question if it comes to mind, and feel distressed if prevented from doing so?
- confess or apologize?

- express concerns about self or others doing the "right" things, adhering to rules?
- worry he or she doesn't believe in God?
- feel distressed about experiencing unwanted sexual or "bad" or scary thoughts, images, or impulses?
- check, repeat, and/or count certain behaviors?
- redo certain behaviors (turning light switches on and off, closing and locking doors, entering and exiting rooms, stepping in certain spots)?
- touch and tap things in particular ways?
- worry about making mistakes in homework?
- hold himself or herself to unrealistic standards and become distressed if falling short?
- study, seek reassurance, or express doubts about performance?
- check backpacks, homework binders, teachers' instructions?
- feel the need to say or do specific things to prevent bad things from happening?

- avoid certain numbers your child believes are "bad" or unlucky?

If you have determined that your child is suffering from OCD, you can follow the steps outlined in this chapter. They are the same steps you learned about in earlier chapters, with two exceptions: (1) you will not teach him to use smart talk, because he could use smart talk as a ritual; and (2) you will do a specific type of exposure—*exposure with response (ritual) prevention* (ERP). All the other principles outlined thus far in this book apply to helping children with OCD. If you completed the worksheets in earlier chapters, you will use that information to complete the Rituals I Do in Trigger Situations Worksheet as well as the Before and After ERP Worksheets.

About ERPs

ERPs are just like the exposures described earlier, except that they are geared toward preventing your child from engaging in rituals while in a trigger situation. British psychologist Victor Meyer developed this treatment in the 1960s, and since then, hundreds of clinical trials have established ERPs as the gold standard of effective treatment for OCD. When doing ERPs, your child will use in vivo and imaginal types of exposures.

Consider twelve-year-old Vince, who engages in symmetry rituals (see table 9). Vince is especially concerned about touch and tactile sensations he experiences throughout the day. He feels the need to touch certain things equally on his left and right sides. He feels distressed, distracted, and tense until he does a ritual to even things up. If he scratches an itch on his right earlobe, he must scratch the other earlobe in exactly the same manner. If he touches a chair with his right hand, he must do the same with his left. As you can imagine, engaging in such rituals all day can be distracting and exhausting. Often Vince chooses to lie or sit completely still so he will not be triggered to do so many rituals.

In an ERP, your child deliberately enters the trigger situation and refrains from engaging in any rituals. An ERP designed for Vince might have him pat his right leg, which would trigger his obsession: *If I leave things uneven, it will bug me so much that I won't be able to focus on anything else.* He would then resist the urge to do the evening ritual of touching his left leg. The goal would be for him to learn that he can do things even if he feels unsettled and preoccupied because he did not do his customary ritual and that he can tolerate any fear, anxiety, or discomfort in the process.

Doing ERPs

Planning ERPs is similar to planning exposures for other anxiety problems (see chapter 8). You will start with the information you already have: your child's trigger situation list, the results of the downward arrow analysis, and the Avoidance and Safety Behaviors I Do with My Child Worksheet.

Step 1. Create a List of Situations that Trigger Obsessions

From the monitoring you have already done, you should have a list of situations that trigger your child's obsessions. Based on this information, you and your child are ready to complete the Rituals I Do in Trigger Situations Worksheet (which you will use instead of the Avoidance and Safety Behaviors I Do in Trigger Situations Worksheet when doing ERPs). You can find a blank copy in appendix I (http://www.newharbinger.com/39539).

Even if you think you and your child already know all the rituals she engages in, I recommend taking the time to go through the list in table 9. Ask your child if she does each ritual. As she describes what she does, consider whether her behavior is *excessive* —does she do this more than an average child of her age? On the worksheet, record her fear thermometer rating for being in the trigger situation while *not* doing the customary ritual.

Now arrange the situations in hierarchical order, with the highest ratings at the top. Here is Vince's list of trigger situations:

- Scratching an itch (6)
- Crossing my leg (5)
- Resting my arm on one side (5)
- Raising my hand (5)
- Hearing a sound on one side (4)
- Seeing something on one side (4)
- Bumping a body part (4)
- Moving an object to one side (3)
- Looking in one direction (2)

Step 2: Select a Situation that Triggers Obsessions, and Identify Sub-situations

As when doing general exposures, I recommend you use the trigger situation with the lowest rating to create your child's first ERP ladder. In Vince's case, that would be looking in one direction. After your child has completed a few ERPs, he will likely have greater confidence and be more willing to take on ERPs with higher degrees of difficulty.

When selecting situations for ERPs, keep in mind that your child's task is to refrain entirely from doing the associated ritual. He can't wait until later to do the ritual, which is the natural temptation. For example, if Vince believes he can do an evening ritual after his ERP of only looking in one direction while refraining from looking in the other direction, he will likely assign a lower fear rating to the ERP experiment than it truly merits, and the exposure will not be effective. When selecting a situation for an ERP, make sure your child knows this. Let's see how Vince and his father selected the situation to use for his first ERP.

Parent: We've filled out the Rituals I Do in Trigger Situations Worksheet and put the situations in order of how challenging they are according to your fear thermometer rating. Are you with me?

Vince: Yes, Dad. Do we start with the one that will be easiest?

Parent: Yes, but if you want to start with a harder one, that's fine, too. Where do you want to start?

Vince: The easiest one for me would be to look in one direction and then not do the ritual of looking in the other direction. Can I start with that?

Parent: Sure! So let's think about how you can do this. For the ERP, you're going to have to look in one direction, wait to feel the urge to do the ritual of making things even by looking in the other direction, and then not do that. Right?

Vince: Yeah, Dad. It is super easy for me to look only one way out of some windows, but I want to look both ways out of others.

Parent: That's interesting. Let's list all the windows and see which will be easiest.

Vince: That's a lot of windows!

Parent: Let's see how many there are. (*Vince and his father walk through their apartment with a pad of paper, stopping first at the window in the kitchen, which faces another building.*) What about this one? How hard do you think it would be to look only to the left and not to the right?

Vince: (*going to the window*) That's no problem, a 1.5 fear thermometer rating.

Parent: Remember, not doing the ritual means not doing it later, either. And not doing it from another location.

Vince: I know. This window is easy because nothing catches my eye. When there is something to look at, it's harder.

Parent: Great! That gives us more information about Worry Dog, too. Now let's try the window by the dining table. Look out in one direction and see what happens.

Vince: (*going to the second window*) This one's much harder. There is a lot to see, so I want to look in both directions. This window would be a 3 or even a 4.

Parent: Good job! Let's go to the balcony. Why don't we see what happens when you stand inside and look through the glass doors?

Vince: Standing here, I can't see much except the sky—so super easy. It's a 1.

Vince and his father visit each window and door in their apartment and rate the following sub-situations for the ERP. Note that some of the sub-situations have higher ratings than the general situation of looking in one direction, which is a 2:

- Standing outside on balcony (4)
- Dining room window (4)
- Living room window (3)
- Parents' bedroom window (2)
- Kitchen window (1.5)
- Vince's bedroom window (1.5)
- Balcony door from inside (1)

Step 3. Create an ERP Exposure Ladder

After you and your child have selected a trigger situation and identified sub-situations, you are ready to plan experiments. Vince's ERP ladder for looking out windows or doors in his apartment while refraining from evening rituals has eight rungs, with fear thermometer ratings from 1 to 4. Vince and his father have the following conversation to plan their experiments:

Parent: Vince, are you ready to sit down with me and plan some ERP experiments for looking out our windows?

Vince: Really? I wanted to chill today.

Parent: I understand. Remember when we talked about rewards for your work conquering your worries?

Vince: Can we go shoot hoops after we do this?

Parent: Sure thing!

Vince: Okay. Let's get this over with! How do we start?

Parent: Let's look at the ladder.

Vince: Well, looking out through the glass doors to the balcony is a 1.

Parent: That might be too easy, but you could start there. Will you be tempted to do the evening ritual?

Vince: Probably a bit. But if I don't do it, I don't think that will bug me too much.

Parent: What might happen?

Vince: I might feel a little weird, I guess.

Parent: Will feeling weird affect anything else? When we did the Downward Arrow Worksheet last week, you said that if you can't do the evening ritual, you sometimes feel preoccupied and worry you won't be able to focus on other things that are important to you.

Vince: Since I can't see anything specific from inside the balcony doors, the urge to look the other way won't be strong. If I feel weird, it won't last long.

Parent: Wait, I just thought of something. Are there any other things you might want to do instead of the evening ritual? Maybe pretend you're doing the ERP and see what comes up.

Vince: Hmm. With a window where I can actually see things, I'd be tempted to view the other side from another window. Like if I did this ERP in your bedroom, I'd want to do the evening ritual in the dining room because it has the same view. I would have to force myself to not look the other way out the dining room window as I walked past it from your room.

Parent: Good job! That sounds like a variation on the evening ritual. We should keep an eye out for that temptation as we plan these experiments. Is it okay if I check with you?

Vince: Sure.

Parent: And you mentioned our bedroom window. That is a 2 on the ladder, so you could plan to do that one next.

Step 4: ERP Role-Play Practice

Before your child runs her first ERP experiment, find ways to practice it. Even if your child thinks practice will be too easy, I recommend you insist on doing it. It never hurts and almost always is helpful. Vince and his father expect his first ERP to be quite easy, but they do a trial run just to be sure their plan doesn't have any issues that need to be addressed. Imaginal ERPs are a useful way for your child to practice ERPs before doing them in real life (in vivo). Help her imagine doing the ERP by narrating to herself (silently or aloud) what she would be thinking, feeling, and sensing in a trigger situation, while refraining from doing rituals.

As with other exposures, practice may elicit a higher than expected fear thermometer rating. Don't worry; this is therapeutic. As you facilitate ERP practice with your child, make it fun and be sure to reward her afterward. Here is the practice Vince did; note that, unlike Vashti and her mother, Vince's father was an observer rather than a participant in the role-play:

Parent: Okay, buddy, before you run your first ERP experiment, let's do a trial run.

Vince: How do we do that?

Parent: You can run the ERP in your imagination. You'll pretend to look out the balcony doors from inside only to the left, resisting the urge to look to the right to even things up. You could do it aloud or in your mind.

Vince: I don't think I need to practice that. It will be too easy!

Parent: So what if it's easy? Then you'll earn a reward for doing nothing.

Doesn't seem like such a bad deal, does it?

Vince: Fine. I'll do it.

Parent: Why don't you stand near where you'll be when you do the actual ERP, so you can feel and hear things that will be there when you do it? Just close your eyes and imagine you are looking left, that you have the urge to look right, but that you do not.

Vince: (*opening his eyes after thirty seconds*) I did it!

Parent: How was it?

Vince: It was harder than I expected.

Parent: What happened?

Vince: I really wanted to do the evening ritual, even in my imagination.

Parent: Did you do it?

Vince: No, Dad. But my fear thermometer rating was more like a 2 or 3 than a 1. I think when I actually do it, it will be a 3.

Parent: That's really good for us to know. Did what you expected happen?

Vince: I felt a little weird, like something was missing.

Parent: Are you okay with that?

Vince: Yes. I feel okay.

Parent: Are you surprised? Did you think the practice would go this way?

Vince: I'm surprised the weird feeling passed so quickly. I thought it would stay and bug me.

Parent: Great work, Vince. Want to go shoot hoops?

Step 5: Running the ERP Experiment

Set up a convenient and consistent time each week that works for both you and your child to review and plan future ERP experiments. After an ERP has been planned and practiced satisfactorily, your child will to do the experiment several times every day. For example, Vince and his father decided Sunday afternoons were a good time for planning and practice. Vince also agreed to do the experiment at least twice a day—once before school and once after coming home from school, as well as on weekends.

Before beginning the experiment, have your child complete the Before ERP Worksheet. You can find a blank copy in appendix J (http://www.newhar binger.com/39539). As with other exposures, if your child doesn't feel highly confident about doing the ERP, as indicated by his response to the last question, consider making it easier. In Vince's case, although his confidence remained high, he and his father upgraded his fear thermometer rating from 1 to 3 after the practice. Here is the worksheet Vince completed with his dad before running his first experiment.

Vince's Before ERP Worksheet

What I plan to do: *Look out toward the balcony and sky or whatever is in one direction and not do my evening ritual of looking in the other direction.*

What am I most worried will happen? *I'll feel weird, like something is missing. It will be on my mind for about 10 minutes. I might not enjoy those minutes as much as if I had just done the ritual.*

How will I know if this happens? *My dad can set a timer for 10 minutes, and we can see how I feel.*

How strongly do I believe my prediction is correct (0–100%)? *95%*

What will my fear thermometer rating be? *3*

Which rituals might I want to do? *I'll want to look in the other direction.*

How confident do I feel that I can do the exposure without doing a ritual? High? Medium? Low? *High*

Immediately after completing the first ERP, facilitate a review of what your child learned by completing the After ERP Worksheet. You can find a blank copy in appendix K (http://www. newharbinger. com/39539). Here is Vince's:

Vince's After ERP Worksheet

Did what I was most worried about occur? Yes or No? *No. I forgot about wanting to do my evening ritual before the timer went off.*

What did happen? Was I surprised? *At first, I felt a 3.5 fear rating, which made me worry I'd feel weird for a long time, but then it went down to a 2 really quickly. I was surprised it went down so quickly. I had fun playing basketball with Dad.*

What was my fear thermometer rating? *3.5 and then a 2*

What did I learn? *I learned that I didn't feel very weird and that I forgot about wanting to even things up more quickly than I expected.*

After the exposure, congratulate, praise, and hug your child. Provide any promised reward.

Step 6. Climbing More Rungs on the ERP Ladder

After your child can do an ERP without doing any rituals, and do so with relative ease, move to the next rung of the ladder. In most cases, each ERP will need to be done several times, though if your child progresses rapidly, there is no need to hold him back, as long as you follow the steps outlined here. In fact, because ERP experiments are most effective when done in a random order, your main concern should be your child's level of motivation. If your child is game to do harder experiments, by all means encourage this.

Vince, for example, chose looking out the dining room window as his second experiment. This was a 4 on the fear thermometer, and thus was not the next rung on the ladder, but Vince wanted to jump to it because he spends so much time in the dining room doing homework and meeting with his tutor. He was tired of being distracted by evening rituals during his studies. The window is large, and many things can catch his eye. In addition, because looking out the balcony doors had been upgraded to a 3, Vince had already successfully moved to a higher level of difficulty, giving him greater confidence. Successfully completing the dining room window exposure would enable him to skip some of the easier exposures, including looking out the kitchen window and his bedroom window.

When your child has completed one entire ERP ladder—hip, hip, hooray! Rewards are in order. And your child is ready to start a new ladder. Go back to your child's situation hierarchy and ask what she wants to tackle next. If she wants to take on a situation that seems like a big jump, that's fine. If she decides to take it a little slower, no harm done. Either way, she knows all the ERP experiments will be run, regardless of how long it takes to plan and implement them.

SUMMARY: What Did You Learn from This Chapter?

- Obsessions are unwanted recurrent worries, thoughts, images, or impulses that engender anxiety, fear, and distress.
- Compulsions (rituals) involve repetitive behaviors or thoughts to suppress or neutralize an obsession, prevent the feared consequences, and reduce distress.
- A special type of exposure called *exposure with response prevention* (ERP) is used to treat OCD.
- In an ERP, your child deliberately enters the situation that triggers his obsessions and refrains from engaging in any rituals.
- The six steps for an ERP are to create a list of the situations that trigger your child's obsessions, select a situation and identify subsituations, create an ERP ladder, practice the first ERP, run that ERP, and climb more rungs on the ladder until complete.

CHAPTER 11

Develop ERPs for OCD

This chapter provides exposure ideas for various types of obsessions. I have not covered every type of obsession, but rather concentrated on those I see most frequently. For each type, I give a general description of the obsession, followed by a brief case as an example. Note that I have only provided the Before ERP Worksheets for each, but your child will also complete the After ERP Worksheet, as you saw in the previous chapter.

Intrusive Thoughts, Images, and Impulses

Even people without an anxiety disorder have unwanted thoughts, images, and impulses, but they dismiss them as unimportant. However, children with obsessions involving intrusive images have great difficulty with these thoughts. They become extremely distressed and engage in rituals to avoid the thoughts or make them go away. The more a child tries to avoid thinking the thought or mitigating the thought by doing neutralizing rituals, the more her mind gets stuck on it.

Intrusive thoughts, images, and impulses can be related to other obsessions the child has. For example, a child who also has aggressive obsessions might experience unwanted, gory images of injury to herself or others, or she might experience the urge to yell profanity or to steal something (with no intention of doing so). Some children, however, experience intrusive thoughts, images, and impulses that are unrelated to other obsessions.

Rituals related to intrusive images, thoughts, or impulses include reassurance seeking; checking; avoidance of movies, newspapers, television, or other media that could trigger the intrusive images; avoidance of situations related to the images or thoughts; and rituals designed to replace the scary image with one that is happier.

It can be difficult or impossible to find a situation in real life that mimics some obsessions. Therefore, imaginal exposures are especially useful for intrusive images. Imaginal exposures were discussed in chapter 8, and the principles are the same when used in ERPs.

Seven-year-old Jamal experiences unwanted images of his dog, Zippy, being hit by a car. This is an aggressive obsession because it involves fear of harm coming to a loved pet, and it also involves unwanted images. The images are vivid and horrifying, and he can't make them stop. He further fears that *because* he is experiencing the images, Zippy is *more likely* to meet this horrible fate. This adds to his distress and exemplifies the magical thinking that is so common with obsessions and compulsions. Jamal's parents have noticed that he engages in several rituals. He checks on Zippy's whereabouts frequently, and he seeks reassurance from his parents regarding Zippy's care while he is at school or involved in other activities. Jamal frequently asks his parents why he has these images: "Is it an omen?" "Why do I keep picturing Zippy being hurt?" "Do you think Zippy will be hit by a car some day?"

As a parent, you may feel hard-pressed to recommend that your child expose himself more to what is distressing, but that is exactly what will get him unstuck and give him relief. Don't forget that if he feels victimized by intrusive thoughts or images, taking charge by exposing himself to them on purpose through ERPs will put him in a position of power. This can be constructive and positive in and of itself.

Jamal and his parents could create an ERP ladder that includes varying degrees of exposure to thoughts of Zippy's demise. Jamal will use imaginal exposures because Zippy is not dead and the situation must be created in Jamal's imagination. When planning imaginal exposures, I tell children that it should be like watching a video in their mind. This type of ERP experiment does not negate the fact that it would be horrible if the feared event ever occurred; rather, it helps the child to stop overvaluing the event and thus remaining stuck on it.

This is the ERP ladder Jamal used, followed by his Before ERP Worksheet:

- Imagine entire image, including all scenes. (10)
- Imagine last scene of the image: "Zippy is badly hurt." (9)
- Imagine third scene: "Zippy is hit by a car." (8)
- Imagine second scene: "Zippy runs into the street." (7)
- Imagine first scene: "Zippy runs out the front door." (5)
- Write the sentence "Zippy gets hit by a car." (4)

Jamal's Before ERP Worksheet

What I plan to do: *Write "Zippy gets hit by a car" twenty-five times a day and keep the sheets of paper out so I see them a lot.*

What am I most worried will happen? *I will worry even more about something happening to Zippy. I'll have a fear rating of at least 4 all day on every day I do this.*

How will I know if this happens? *I will tell Mom and Dad my fear rating at the end of the day.*

How strongly do I believe my prediction is correct (0–100%)? *60%*

What will my fear thermometer rating be? *4–5*

Which rituals might I want to do? *Check to see where Zippy is. Always want to know where he is.*

How confident do I feel that I can do the exposure without doing avoidance or safety behaviors? High? Medium? Low? *High*

Perfectionistic Obsessions

Obsessions can take the form of excessive worry about the possibility of failing to meet self-imposed standards or goals. These obsessions are referred to as "perfectionistic obsessions." Joseph (who was introduced in chapter 1) and Camilla (chapter 4) have perfectionistic obsessions. I see a high percentage of children (and adults) who suffer from these types of obsessions. (Note that some children have perfectionistic worries but engage in avoidance and safety behaviors rather than rituals; we say they have generalized anxiety disorder, not OCD.)

Many of these children are not appropriately diagnosed and treated because they appear to be "model" children. They get great grades, engage in all the "right" activities, and are adored by teachers for their dedication to their studies. Although these children suffer a great deal on the inside, the disadvantages of their obsessions often come to light only when they become severe. Nevertheless, even obsessions with moderate levels of severity can exact high costs on the sufferer.

Remember—all obsessions exist on a continuum. A moderate amount of drive can help us achieve great results. It motivates us to do our best—an excellent job—given the resources we have (such as time and energy). An excellent job is not, however, a perfect job. Perfection is not a realistic, achievable goal in most human pursuits. Nevertheless, a child with a perfectionistic obsession believes she can—and, in fact, must—meet these unrealistic standards. But unrealistic standards simply can't be met. This is why these children often feel they are never doing well enough.

Another reason perfectionistic obsessions are challenging to manage is that they have overtly positive results for the sufferer: good grades, accolades from teachers and parents, and a sense of future success in this increasingly competitive world. These obsessions come with built-in reinforcements from many sources in the child's world. Furthermore, individuals with perfectionistic obsessions tend to have less self-awareness than do those suffering from other types of obsessions. A child with perfectionistic obsessions is more likely than a child with a contamination obsession to believe her obsession.

Some rituals associated with perfectionistic obsessions are obvious to parents. Over-studying, schedule checking, use of special pens, backpack checking, and excessively seeking reassurance that assignments were done properly all clearly reflect a measurable perfectionistic standard. Other compulsions, however, are more difficult to detect. For example, your child may worry about seemingly inconsequential decisions, such as what to order at a restaurant or what color T-shirt to buy on vacation. The feared consequence in such situations is usually that the child will not make the best decision.

Children with perfectionistic obsessions often resort to rituals such as asking others to make decisions for them, seeking consensus, avoiding making decisions, and optimizing in their mind (spending lots of time thinking through all possible outcomes so they can be certain that whatever they choose is best). I once worked with an eight-year-old boy whose parents thought he was seriously depressed because he refused to do things he had previously enjoyed and never seemed to feel satisfied with his efforts at sports or school, despite his considerable ability and accomplishments. When he was successfully treated for perfectionistic obsessions, his parents realized his problem was not actually depression.

Other rituals I see children use include quitting an activity or sport when their performance is not stellar, saying they no longer like doing something when perfect performance cannot be achieved, refusing to play a game due to fear of losing, and constantly checking the clock due to fears of being late and missing something. Procrastination is another common ritual. Though some children with this obsession rush to get their work done for fear they won't have time to complete it and double-check everything, others procrastinate because they anticipate the excessive amount of time and energy the rituals they do require.

Joseph, the twelve-year-old from chapter 1, provides an example of perfectionistic obsessions. The rituals he does include spending excessive amounts of time on homework and over-preparing or over-studying. He always does his homework immediately after school and avoids activities that might interfere with doing it, such as getting together with friends. He asks his mother or father to quiz him even when he knows the material. He seeks reassurance by telling them he thinks he hasn't studied enough for a test. He repeatedly checks his planner to be sure he didn't miss an assignment and checks to see if his homework really is in his backpack.

A conversation between Joseph and his mother about creating ERPs might sound like this:

Parent: Joe, you know how we've been talking about helping you develop strategies to reduce your stress about schoolwork and stuff?

Joseph: Yeah.

Parent: Well, I think you're ready to take some next steps.

Joseph: Mom, I'm fine the way things are. I like being busy all the time.

Parent: I understand you feel that way right now. But we've been talking about the big spikes of worry you have. You seem unhappy at those times.

Joseph: You're right. I wish I didn't stress out so much.

Parent: That's why we are working this program.

Joseph: I know, I know. Okay, what's the next step?

Parent: The next step is to set up some ERP ladders so you can practice doing what triggers you without doing the rituals you usually do. Could we look at your trigger situation list and figure out which rituals you do in each of the situations?

Joseph: What does ERP stand for?

Parent: Exposure with response prevention. Remember we talked about the worry hill and trying to fill your brain with more green candies? You want to get to the other side of the hill, where you can be in the situation and not feel so stressed. To do that, you have to practice being in the situation lots of times without doing the behaviors you usually do. Every time you practice being in the situation and don't do any rituals, you can add a green candy to your brain.

Joseph: I kind of remember. What exactly do I have to do?

Parent: Joe, it's not a matter of what you *have* to do. It's a matter of using proven tools to help you feel less worried.

Joseph: I see what you mean. So what do we do now?

Parent: Could we look at that trigger situation list together?

Joseph: Sure. Where is it?

Parent: I have it right here. Why don't you take a quick look at it before we get started?

Joseph: Okay. (*He looks at the list.*) I remember all this from last week.

Parent: Great. Let's read through it together to make sure it's still accurate and complete. (*She reads aloud the list, along with the fear thermometer ratings Joseph has given.*)

Joseph: That sounds right.

Parent: Let's look at the list of rituals you do when you are in these situations. I have it right here. Can we read through it together? We need to consider other rituals besides avoiding being in the situation.

Joseph: Okay. (*They go through the list of rituals.*)

Parent: Let's start with the situations with the lowest fear thermometer ratings and see which rituals you tend to do in them. Which situations have the lowest ratings?

Joseph: Going out to dinner on a school night. But it depends on the restaurant and how much homework I have. If I finish all my homework before dinner, then it's not a problem to go out, unless I have music to practice afterward. Also, if I'm working on a long-term project, it's hard for me to go out.

Parent: Your fear rating does go up or down according to different situations. Good for you for noticing that! Let's put a rung on your ERP ladder for going out to dinner on school nights that won't be higher than a 4 on your fear thermometer.

Joseph: I'm usually okay when we go to Quikway, because it's faster than eating dinner at home. El Molino takes longer because we always run into people you and Dad know, and you want to talk and talk. So I get a higher fear rating there. Going to Grandma's also takes way too long. I for sure do all of my homework early if I know we're going to Grandma's.

Parent: Good observations. We can use all this information to plan ERP experiments.

Joseph: Sounds good to me.

Parent: What would your rating be if we went to Quikway on a night when you have choir practice after school and lots of homework to do after dinner?

Joseph: I wouldn't want to go out under those circumstances. But if I had to? A 5.

Parent: What about if you had a medium amount of homework?

Joseph: A 4.

Parent: And if you had choir after school and only twenty minutes of homework left?

Joseph: 2.

Parent: Now let's use the same details, except that on these rungs it will be going to Grandma's for dinner. What would your fear rating be to go to Grandma's if you had lots of homework and didn't do any of it before going? Doing homework early is one of the rituals on your list.

Joseph: That would be an 8.

Parent: Okay, good. What about if you had a medium amount of work and didn't do it before going?

Joseph: 6.

Parent: And if you had just twenty minutes of homework and went to Grandma's?

Joseph: 4.

Parent: What makes it a 4?

Joseph: I could miss something and have more homework than I thought. That's why I always check to be sure. If I'm not home, I can't check. That means I'll be nervous until I get home and can check.

Parent: So checking is another ritual?

Joseph: I guess so. I do it automatically when I'm at home.

Parent: It's good you noticed that, Joe. Good job! Let's write checking on your rituals list. What do you think about doing an experiment at El Molino? It takes more time than Quikway, but less than Grandma's.

Joseph: El Molino would be about a 5, but if you and Dad started talking to your friends, it would go higher.

Parent: I've noticed how irritable you get when we do that. Remember last time when we ran into the Worths? You got into trouble with Dad and me because you badgered us to leave so much we couldn't enjoy our conversation with them.

Joseph: I know. Sorry.

Parent: That's water under the bridge, but do you think we should put badgering on the list of rituals?

Joseph: I guess so. I get worried and want to get home to finish my work.

Parent: I know you do. But you and I both know the badgering behavior just feeds Worry Wart.

Based on this conversation, Joseph and his mother developed the following ERP ladder:

- Going to Grandma's for dinner when I have lots of homework (8)
- Going to El Molino when I have lots of homework (7–8)
- Going to Grandma's for dinner with a medium amount of homework (6)
- Going to El Molino with a medium amount of homework (5–6)
- Going to Quikway when I have lots of homework (5)
- Going to Grandma's for dinner with a little homework (4)
- Going to El Molino with a little homework (3–4)
- Going to Quikway with a medium amount of homework (3)
- Going to Quikway with a little homework (2)

Joseph would likely start his first ERP by going to Quikway on a school night when he has about twenty minutes of homework to complete after dinner. Here is his Before ERP Worksheet:

Joseph's Before ERP Worksheet

What I plan to do: *Go out to dinner at Quikway this Tuesday night without finishing all of my homework first. I will save my math for after dinner.*

What am I most worried will happen? *It will take a long time to get our dinner—more than twenty-five minutes—and I will feel super worried. I may not feel like eating much. I won't want to talk or waste time. I'll get annoyed with my parents if they are taking too long.*

How will I know if this happens? *I can see if I feel nervous. I can see if I don't finish my food. If Mom and Dad tell me to relax, which they do when I'm acting annoyed with them.*

How strongly do I believe my prediction is correct (0–100%)? *60%*

What will my fear thermometer rating be? *3*

> **Which rituals might I want to do?** *I will want to remind them to hurry up. I'll check my watch the entire time and tell Mom and Dad what time it is.*
>
> **How confident do I feel that I can do the exposure without doing avoidance or safety behaviors? High? Medium? Low?** *High*

Contamination Obsessions

Children with contamination obsessions worry they (or loved ones, or both) will come in contact with germs, dirt, toxins, or broken glass and become ill or harmed in some way. Rituals associated with contamination obsessions typically involve excessive washing or cleaning, as well as attempts to avoid "unclean" or "unsafe" environments or objects throughout the course of the day.

When treating a child with a contamination obsession, I like to use a feather duster in ERPs. The child uses the feather duster to collect "germs" or "yuck" and then "contaminates" himself by dusting his hands and body, belongings, clothes, towels, and so on. This is effective because it rapidly teaches the child that although he is constantly exposed to the contaminant, the feared consequences don't happen and that he can manage the uncertainty that they might happen. Sometimes I make a small, portable feather duster out of a piece of cotton cord, with one end frayed, that a child can use on trips or at school. The child can carry it in his pocket or backpack.

The feather duster technique is effective because it eliminates the confusing practice of trying to prevent your child from washing his hands at particular times or doing other rituals (avoiding dirt, excessive laundering). As he progresses through feather duster ERPs, his washing and other rituals will be automatically reduced because he knows he will simply be re-contaminated after washing.

Individuals with contamination obsessions often like to keep particular spaces, such as a bedroom, safe from contaminants. This is problematic because it only defers the issue. A child can avoid difficulty during the day because he expects to shower and enter the germfree safe space at the end of the day. Using a feather duster eliminates this ritual because it contaminates everything.

If your child rates all the trigger situations for the feather duster higher than a 4, he may use a tissue to touch the contaminated surface and then feather dust the tissue. This typically lowers his fear rating because less of the contaminant is perceived to be on the duster. If you run into this issue, don't be deterred. Calmly let him know you have a solution. Ask, "What would your fear thermometer rating be if you touched a tissue to the doorknob and then feather dusted the tissue?" Sometimes a child will want one tissue and then another tissue and then the feather duster to get his rating to a 4 or below. It doesn't matter. All that matters is that he does not avoid doing the ERP altogether.

As your child uses the dusting technique daily, track his fear thermometer rating. Find a time of day that works for both of you and that isn't stressful or busy, and ask how his fear thermometer is tracking. Be sure he completes an After Exposure Worksheet so he can focus on the lessons learned from being exposed to feared contaminants 24/7. Praise and reward him for doing the feather duster ERPs. He needs to continue dusting until he feels comfortable being exposed to whatever is on the feather duster at any given time. After mastering this ERP, he can advance to the next rung on the ladder—or skip to a higher rung—and pick a new contaminant to feather dust.

Not all children with contamination obsessions worry about being harmed by the contaminants. Sometimes it's just the yuck factor. In that case, your child may not fear specific consequences but may worry about being preoccupied with having yuck on her. The feared consequence of knowing that yuck is on her usually involves worries that the preoccupation will be distressing, interfere with feeling at peace, or get in the way of focusing on more important things.

Some children with contamination obsessions worry about spreading germs to others. These children fear feeling responsible for negatively affecting a loved one. The following feather duster ERP ladder was made by eleven-year-old Alisha, who isn't worried about harm to herself, but fears spreading contaminants to family members, particularly her baby brother. The rituals she does include avoiding touching her family members, showering and bathing excessively, hand washing, using hand sanitizer, and seeking reassurance from her parents.

The following ERP ladder entails Alisha using a feather duster to grab germs from various trigger items and then contaminating her family or items they touch. All the rungs require Alisha to contaminate her personal and family items.

- Use the duster on the flusher on a school toilet (10)
- Use the duster on the toilet paper dispenser by a school toilet (10)
- Use the duster on a bathroom stall door and latch at school (9)

- Use the duster on desks in class deemed most yucky (9)
- Use the duster on a classroom doorknob (8)
- Use the duster on a restaurant restroom doorknob (7–10)
- Use the duster on a coffee shop counter (5)
- Use the duster on a grocery cart handle (5)
- Use the duster on old paper money or coins (4)
- Use the duster on chairs in a classroom (4)
- Use the duster on the outside doorknob of our house (2)

Alisha agreed to start with dusting the outside doorknob of their house because it had the lowest rating. Here is Alisha's Before ERP Worksheet:

Alisha's Before ERP Worksheet

What I plan to do: *Feather dust the doorknob of our house on both sides and then dust my brother's toys and high chair, our table, the dishes, the forks and knives, my room, me, my clothes. Every time I wash my* hands or shower, or after the dishes come out of the dishwasher, I will dust again so I know germs are everywhere.

What am I most worried will happen? *I worry my brother will get sick and need to go to the hospital. I won't be able to think of other things until I know for sure he's not sick. I won't do as good a job on my homework. I won't be able to sleep. I'll worry all day at school about making sure he isn't sick when I get home.*

How will I know if this happens? *If my brother gets sick, I'll know it, and if he goes to the hospital, that will be obvious. My teacher will ask why I did a bad job on my homework. I can tell Mom or Dad how I slept and that the only thing I thought about at school was my brother.*

How strongly do I believe my prediction is correct (0–100%)? *40%*

What will my fear thermometer rating be? *2*

> **Which rituals might I want to do?** *Since washing will do no good, I will want to watch my brother for signs he is getting sick. I will want to ask Mom to take his temperature and ask her if she thinks he might be sick.*
>
> **How confident do I feel that I can do the exposure without doing avoidance or safety behaviors? High? Medium? Low?** *High*

Aggressive Obsessions

Aggressive obsessions involve fears of harming oneself, harm coming to oneself, or harming someone else. Of course, most of us have had passing thoughts such as *What if I ran my bike off the road?* or *What if I got so angry that I pushed that person off the balcony?* or *What if a kid in woodshop hits me with a hammer by accident?* Children with aggressive obsessions get stuck on these thoughts and impulses and fear the behavior manifested in the thought will occur. They may fear they will unintentionally lose control and hurt either themselves or someone else, or that harm will be done to them.

Many children suffering from this type of obsession believe that having a thought or impulse is equivalent to doing something harmful or makes them more likely to actually do it. Of course, being stuck on such a thought is extremely distressing, so they engage in rituals that help them feel more certain no harm will occur. Such rituals include seeking reassurance, checking, and avoidance (staying away from balconies, not handling knives or scissors, and being excessively cautious in feared situations).

Some children have aggressive obsessions that are less alarming than others. For example, a child might simply fear bumping into someone (perhaps while riding a bike or running) and hence causing harm. Rituals associated with such a fear include avoidance of certain situations or of physical contact with other children, overly cautious behaviors, and excessively checking the well-being of a child who was accidentally bumped.

Other children fear they might harm themselves or commit suicide. This will most certainly give a parent pause. In such a case, your child must be assessed for suicide risk by a mental health professional. If OCD is diagnosed, then you can follow the guidelines presented in this book. Understand that children with aggressive obsessions are neither suicidal nor homicidal. They do not want to harm themselves or others, but are afraid they might. Nor do they exhibit symptoms of severe depression, anger, or other acting-out behaviors. Because the content of some aggressive obsessions can be alarming, you may think it would be easier for a seasoned CBT specialist to manage. However, in general, aggressive obsessions are no more difficult to treat than other obsessions, and they are not more serious than others. The content is just scarier.

Farron is a ten-year-old who loves soccer and many other sports. She is a super student, has a loving and supportive family and many friends, and overall reports feeling content. At age eight, she began to experience episodes during which she became preoccupied with the possibility that she could or did hurt another child while playing soccer, riding her bike, or playing on the playground. During these episodes, Farron sought reassurance from her parents excessively and apologized to other kids excessively. She was also observed holding back in sports and play. Her parents thought she was a just a caring, sensitive, and empathetic child. These episodes waxed and waned; they didn't disrupt Farron's life until this year, when soccer became more physical and her coaches and teammates urged her to play more aggressively.

Farron's rituals include holding back from putting in her best effort in sports and playing soccer in an overly cautious manner. She always checks to see if she has injured someone and repeatedly asks, "Are you okay?" if she fears she hurt someone. She also rides her bike in an overly careful way when riding with others. She seeks reassurance from her parents and from peers.

This ERP ladder for Farron is a good example of how to construct exposures for aggression obsessions:

- Do a shoulder tackle to gain possession of the ball during a game without asking, "Are you okay?" or checking the girl's condition (8–10)
- Do a shoulder tackle to gain possession of the ball during practice without asking, "Are you okay?" or checking the girl's condition (7)
- Take the ball away from an opponent at a game without asking, "Are you okay?" or checking her condition (6–8)
- Show 100 percent effort and conviction in soccer practice without asking, "Are you okay?" or checking anyone's condition (5–7)
- Take the ball away from a teammate with conviction at practice without asking, "Are you okay?" or checking her condition (5)

Here is Farron's Before ERP Worksheet:

Farron's Before ERP Worksheet

What I plan to do: *Take the ball away from another girl in practice. I will try really hard to get the ball and won't hold back because I don't want to hurt her.*

What am I most worried will happen? *I will hurt whomever I took the ball away from.*

How will I know if this happens? *She will fall down on the field, and maybe an ambulance will come.*

How strongly do I believe my prediction is correct (0–100%)? *20%. I know it probably won't really happen, but it might.*

What will my fear thermometer rating be? *5*

Which rituals might I want to do? *Hold back. Not really try my best to get the ball. Ask if she's okay after I get the ball. Watch her afterward to make sure she's okay.*

How confident do I feel that I can do the exposure without doing avoidance or safety behaviors? High? Medium? Low? *High*

Health-Related Obsessions

Health-related obsessions involve fears about contracting a serious disease or developing a debilitating condition. While no one wants to get sick, children with this obsession are consumed by the fear of it happening. They may worry about things that are unlikely to occur, such as a child having a heart attack. Minor symptoms may become exaggerated, such as worrying that a headache is a sign of a brain tumor.

Nine-year-old Fred has health-related obsessions that are triggered when he hears about other people contracting illnesses. He recently became triggered in social studies when the class studied the bubonic plague and he learned it still exists in remote areas. He also learned about the mumps, measles, and leprosy. Because Fred wants certainty that he won't contract a serious disease, he engages in compulsions, such as searching the Internet for information about diseases and where outbreaks have occurred, and by repeatedly seeking reassurance from his parents: "How do people get the plague?" "Who was the last person in this country to get it?" "Do you think there could be another breakout?"

The following ERP ladder was constructed for Fred's obsession about the plague. The ratings for each rung reflect what he would feel when exposed to this health-related situation without doing his rituals of seeking reassurance and doing Internet research.

- Say the phrase "I can't be 100% sure I won't get the plague." (10)
- View photographs of individuals who have the plague. (9)
- Read a description of the plague. (8)
- Say aloud, "I could get the plague." (6)
- Write the word "plague." (4)
- Say the word "plague" over and over. (3)

In this case, Fred's first ERP would likely be to say aloud the word "plague" repeatedly while refraining from any rituals until his fear thermometer rating reduces significantly. Here is his Before ERP Worksheet:

Fred's Before ERP Worksheet

What I plan to do: *Say the word "plague" 20 times a day.*

What am I most worried will happen? *I will worry more about getting sick. I sort of think that just saying it will make it happen. I could end up getting the plague. I worry so much that I don't want to go out and play after school. I think about it at school, so I can't do all my work.*

How will I know if this happens? *If I get the plague, I will get a fever and a bad headache all of a sudden. My fingers and toes will turn black. I'll need to go to the hospital. I will know I'm worrying if I stay inside after school and not even want to play with Marco. My teacher can tell you if I didn't do all my work.*

How strongly do I believe my prediction is correct (0–100%)? *20% for getting the plague and 60% for worrying about it and not playing outside or doing my schoolwork.*

What will my fear thermometer rating be? *3–4*

Which rituals might I want to do? *Check my forehead for fever;*

> *ask Mom to take my temperature; look at my fingers and toes.*
>
> **How confident do I feel that I can do the exposure without doing avoidance or safety behaviors? High? Medium? Low?** *High*

"Just-So," Ordering and Arranging, and Incompleteness Obsessions

Children with "just-so" and similar kinds of obsessions feel extreme distress when they cannot do things in a particular way, cannot order or arrange things in a preferred manner, or must leave things unfinished or incomplete. They engage in rituals that involve arranging or doing things in particular ways or making movements in a set way. For example, your child might feel the need to adjust how she holds a pencil until it feels just right. She may insist on finishing every step of a ritual without interruption, and if interrupted, may feel the need to restart it from the beginning.

The objects and behaviors of concern to these children may vary, but they carry personal significance for each child. Thus, these obsessions often do not make logical sense to observers. Objects of concern may include toys, bookshelves, desks, drawers, or closets. The behaviors may include modes of dressing and grooming (hair style, type of clothing). A child with one highly specific type of obsession may not be bothered by a different type. For example, if your child has an ordering obsession, he may become upset when a friend innocently disturbs the order of toys in his room, but he may not have any anxiety about the order of things elsewhere. He may not care if his backpack or shoes are muddy, or if a friend's room is in disarray.

Six-year-old Hwan experiences just-so, ordering, and incompleteness obsessions. His rituals include keeping his plastic brick models in a particular order on a specific shelf and completing any model without stopping, even for a brief break. He avoids having friends over because he doesn't want them to "mess up stuff." If anyone does, he becomes distressed and angry. His parents observe that he delays playing in order to finish what he's doing and becomes argumentative when forced to leave a task unfinished. This is the ERP ladder Hwan used.

- Invite friends over to play with my plastic brick models (10)
- Allow my older brother to touch brick models and move them a tiny bit (9)
- Leave building bricks on the floor partially assembled (7)
- Leave five items on my model shelf in the "wrong" order (7)
- Place models on my desk in no order (6)
- Leave a model half-finished for an entire day (6)
- Leave a model half-finished for an hour (4)

Here is his Before ERP Worksheet:

Hwan's Before ERP Worksheet

What I plan to do: *Leave my pencil sharpener out on my desk. Move it around a little every day in a way that it bugs me to see it.*

What am I most worried will happen? *It will bother me when I see it. I might have a hard time falling sleep because I'll know it's sitting there.*

How will I know if this happens? *I will have a high fear thermometer rating, especially at first. I can tell Mom or Dad in the morning if I thought about the pencil sharpener while I was in bed.*

How strongly do I believe my prediction is correct (0–100%)? *70%*

What will my fear thermometer rating be? *3*

Which rituals might I want to do? *Put the pencil sharpener away. Avoid looking at it so it doesn't bug me.*

How confident do I feel that I can do the exposure without doing avoidance or safety behaviors? High? Medium? Low? *High*

Tips and Troubleshooting: Issues While Doing ERPs

Here are some principles to make your child's work with ERPs more effective.

What if my child does not seem ready to move up her ERP ladder?

As with other types of exposures, lack of progress with ERPs can be the result of new or continued avoidance behaviors or rituals. Ask yourself the following questions to determine what is affecting her progress.

Is my child engaging in avoidance? If your child is doing enough ERPs, she may be introducing avoidance behaviors. For example, some children game the system by reporting fear ratings that are higher than they truly experience so they can avoid the exposures they fear most. As you examine the possibility of avoidance, it is important to maintain an objective, neutral attitude about your child's ERP work. Don't let frustration or anger interfere.

Is my child engaging in rituals or creating new rituals during ERPs? Check in with your child about how well she is resisting the urge to engage in rituals. A simple, straightforward, and factual approach is most productive. The following dialogue between John and his mother provides a model.

Parent: Hey, John, can we check in on your ERPs? How are they going?

John: Fine, Mom.

Parent: That's good. How many did you do today? I think you agreed to do three today?

John: I didn't get to them yet.

Parent: Okay. When are you planning to do them?

John: I'm not sure. I don't like doing them.

Parent: I know they're not easy. Nobody finds them comfortable or enjoyable.

But people do them so they can conquer their worries. Like we've been talking about and doing with this program.

John: I'm not sure why I feel this way.

Parent: Maybe we can figure out what's getting in the way. Do you think maybe we made them too hard?

John: No, that's not it. They aren't that hard.

Parent: Hmm. Maybe you're not doing enough of them to get to the other side of the worry hill, and so you are discouraged?

John: Until yesterday I was doing them like I agreed.

Parent: Do you think you might be doing new rituals? The author of the book says some people come up with new rituals during ERPs. Do you have any ideas?

John: I don't think that's happening.

Parent: Let's walk through the last ERP you did. Can you tell me what you did and what you were thinking?

John: I used the feather duster from the toilet paper holder in the restaurant bathroom on myself. I did it like always.

Parent: Were you thinking anything?

John: I told myself after I dusted myself that the germs on the duster aren't that bad—only clean and healthy people go to that restaurant. That kind of stuff. I tried to be reasonable about it.

Parent: I think I know the problem! I'm pretty sure you were reassuring yourself, which is a ritual.

John: I thought it was only reassurance if I asked you.

Parent: No, if you reassure yourself, it has the same effect.

John: Really?

Parent: Yes. Apparently it's pretty common. Do you think you could resist the urge to reassure yourself?

John: I guess? But it happens so automatically.

Parent: They say that when these rituals pop into your head, you can deal with them by telling yourself, *The damage is done* or *Reassuring myself won't help.*

How do I set reasonable goals for my child?

Children with perfectionistic and other obsessions often spend excessive amounts of time completing tasks due to checking, rereading, and needing an overly meticulous process and pace in general. Planning ERPs for such children can involve completing tasks within a reasonable time frame.

The *reasonable person standard* is a legal term referring to behavior that most people regard as normal or acceptable in a given situation. I sometimes use this term with children who have developed rituals that are long-standing and who have lost sight of what is reasonable in their daily activities. The longer your child has been performing rituals, the more likely his view of what is reasonable has become skewed. Reestablishing behaviors that align with a reasonable person standard is a useful goal that most children will accept and embrace. You should be careful, however, that your child doesn't think the standard implies he is no longer reasonable. Use the standard in a positive and helpful manner.

Setting ERP goals for perfectionistic and other obsessions involves establishing reasonable amounts of time for studying and other daily tasks. Ask your child how much time he needs to do something, and have him agree to adhere to it. Children with perfectionistic standards are usually able to accurately estimate about how long a task will take. They run into trouble later, when they begin to doubt themselves or their abilities or think they missed something important. Other ways to establish reasonable time limits are to consult with your child's teacher or have him ask fellow students how much time is spent on a task.

Maintaining a reasonable balance in life that includes academic, social, athletic, and community-based activities can protect your child from the negative impact of perfectionistic and other obsessions. A child fully engaged in activities that are reasonable and appropriate will have less time to engage in rituals; as a result, he will gain general psychological benefits, such as mood regulation and social support, and be more motivated to conquer his anxiety.

SUMMARY: What Did You Learn from This Chapter?

- ERPs for perfectionistic obsessions involve resisting the urge to engage in checking, over-preparing, reassurance seeking, and avoidance rituals while in trigger situations. Use the reasonable person standard to establish time limits for ERPs.

- In ERPs for contamination obsessions, a feather duster is used to gather germs and "yuck" and to contaminate the child as well as objects he touches, both before and after any washing, cleaning, or avoiding rituals.
- ERPs for aggressive obsessions involve resisting doing rituals such as checking for harm done, seeking reassurance, and being overly cautious in trigger situations.
- ERPs targeting health-related obsessions involve resisting engaging in rituals such as reassurance seeking, Internet searches, and excessive visits to the pediatrician.
- ERPs for intrusive thoughts, images, and impulses use imaginal exposures while the child resists doing any rituals.
- ERPs for just-so, ordering and arranging, and incompleteness obsessions involve resisting doing rituals aimed at putting things back in a desired order or manner.

CHAPTER 12

Recognize Progress and Prevent Relapse

As you and your child work through this program, you will notice progress in many ways. Your child may seem less fearful in what were previously distressing situations. He may appear freer and more joyful in daily life. However, your subjective observations are not enough. You should track his progress in eliminating avoidance and safety behaviors and doing exposures and ERPs, as well as your own progress in reducing participation in avoidance and safety behaviors. The following are ways to track his progress and ensure continued mastery of anxiety symptoms.

Daily Observations

I recommend daily observations of the following:
• Is your child relying on avoidance and safety behaviors less?

- Is your child making good progress on his or her exposure ladders?
- Are you reducing your participation in avoidance and safety behaviors?

Weekly Check-Ins

Weekly check-ins with your child are an important part of the process. If he knows you will follow up each week, he is more likely to persevere with the program. Weekly check-ins hold both of you accountable, and he will gain a sense of security and trust in the process if you assess progress regularly. You can find a blank Weekly Check-In Worksheet in appendix L (http://www.newharbinger.com/39539).

I suggest establishing a consistent day of the week for a fifteen-to twenty-minute check-in. Make it a pleasant and rewarding experience for your child. You might talk at a local café over cocoa and a cookie on Sunday afternoons. During this meeting, go over the numbers (number of exposures run, changes in fear thermometer ratings) rather than relying on subjective assessments. Concentrate on the exposure or ERP ladder he is currently tackling, as well as review his current avoidance and safety behaviors list and rituals list and your own avoidance and safety behaviors list. Start by reviewing with him the worksheets he has most recently completed. Stress what he has learned from doing exposures—verbalizing these lessons helps to consolidate the new learning. If he has not started exposures—if you're working instead on naming the fear or tracking parent and child participation in avoidance and safety behaviors—assess progress in these areas.

I find that children are often surprised at their progress. Seeing concrete evidence of mastery can be empowering. These assessments allow you to recognize your child's hard work. Note each and every reduction and praise, congratulate, and reward him for his hard work. The pace of his progress is not as important as consistent movement toward goals. Weekly check-ins also allow for troubleshooting if he runs into challenges.

After recognizing progress during these meetings, you and your child decide as a team which challenges he is ready to take on next. Is it time for the next rung on the exposure ladder? Does he wish to take on more challenging ERPs by skipping a couple rungs? Perhaps he has completed an entire ladder and is ready for another.

The following dialogue is an example of a check-in between Vashti and her mother.

Parent: Vashti, I'm so proud of you for working on your worries with me.

Vashti: Yeah, Mom. Thanks.

Parent: Let's look at how things are going. I've got your exposure ladder, along with your list of avoidance and safety behaviors and my list of avoidance and safety behaviors I do with you.

Vashti: Sounds good.

Parent: First, here's your exposure ladder. Greeting kids with eye contact and saying hi is what you were working on this week, right?

Vashti: Yeah. I think I did pretty well.

Parent: Great! Let's start by seeing how you did with reducing safety behaviors. You agreed to work on not acting busy, pretending not to see other kids, and avoiding eye contact. How did it go?

Vashti: Pretty well!

Parent: That's great to hear. Let's see how we can measure this. Out of ten times that you passed kids in the halls, during recesses, and before and after school, how many times were you able to refrain from those behaviors?

Vashti: I stopped acting busy when I wasn't really busy almost all of the time. I'd say eight out of ten times.

Parent: I'm impressed! What have you learned from this?

Vashti: I thought I'd be forced to talk to everyone if I didn't act busy. But it didn't seem like they noticed. They didn't try to talk a lot to me, like I worried they would.

Parent: Super. So it sounds like that surprised you.

Vashti: Yes, a lot. (*She smiles.*)

Parent: Excellent work, Vashti! I see on your Avoidance and Safety Behaviors I Do in Trigger Situations Worksheet that you estimated your fear rating would be about a 4 for not acting busy? Was that the case?

Vashti: At first it was a 4, maybe even a 4.5. But after I realized kids didn't notice me, it went down to a 2. Each day it got easier. Now it's a 0.

Parent: That is so cool! And you did it all yourself.

Vashti and her mother would continue to assess her progress in relinquishing the behaviors of avoiding eye contact and pretending not to see other children. Then they would talk about the exposure experiment Vashti was currently running: saying hi with eye contact to children she knows but does not know well enough to feel at ease with. Their dialogue might continue as follows.

Parent: Let's look at the experiment you have been running. (*She pulls out the Before Exposure Worksheet.*) Under "What I plan to do," you wrote, "Say hi with eye contact to four kids each day."

Vashti: Most days, I did that.

Parent: That's great! Do you remember everyone you said hi to? That's twenty kids!

Vashti: It didn't seem like that many. (*She smiles.*) But since you added it up, I'd say it was a bit less. But close to twenty.

Parent: The exact number doesn't matter. What's important is that you did it. But it's good to know so we can track your progress, and you can see how well you're doing.

Vashti: Thanks, Mom.

Parent: What have you learned from saying hi with eye contact to kids you don't know very well?

Vashti: They just say hi back. It's no big deal.

Parent: So, you learned...?

Vashti: I learned it's easier than I thought.

Parent: That's a good thing to learn.

Vashti: For sure. Now I don't feel so stressed when I'm walking around or during recess.

Next, with your child, go through all her other avoidance and safety behaviors to see if she has decreased using them and if it has gotten easier to do so. Review her fear thermometer ratings for this week and compare them with her ratings from last week. Make special notes to your child of any reductions you observe. Date the new numbers so you can keep accurate track of progress. Show her the numbers. This is powerful feedback that can keep her motivation strong.

Finally, during this check-in, enlist your child's assistance in rating your progress in reducing your participation in avoidance and safety behaviors. If your goal was to stop providing reassurance and explanation in a particular situation, restate your goal aloud and ask, "How did I do?" You will be surprised at how honest and constructive your child can be in giving feedback. Also ask her what she learned from doing without your accommodating behaviors. Did she feel okay with your reduced participation? Was it as hard as anticipated? Or easier?

Finally, review her fear thermometer ratings. Were her predictions accurate? Too high? Too low? Thank her for the thoughtful feedback. It is important that she knows that you value her feedback and that you are working as a team.

Assess Your Own Progress

In addition to discussing your own participation with your child during the weekly check-in, conduct a careful self-assessment of your performance regarding safety behaviors, rituals, and any ways you enable him to avoid the situations he fears. Consult the list you created on the Avoidance and Safety Behaviors I Do with My Child Worksheet.

- How are you doing?
- If you are struggling in a particular area, what makes it challenging for you?
- Is it difficult when your child shows distress or anger?

Determine what, if anything, is getting in your way, and come up with a solution. Perhaps, for example, you need to play tag team with your child's other parent and assign him or her the responsibility of managing a particular situation with your child.

Maintaining Mental Fitness and Preventing Relapse

Progress is not always linear. Your child may hit snags or even take steps backward along the way. Relapse means your child has gone back to engaging in many or all of his avoidance and safety behaviors or rituals. You, too, can relapse by returning to your prior behaviors. In either case, your child will experience increased anxiety.

I have incorporated the most up-to-date information about how to ensure success and reduce the chance of relapse into this program. As I explained in chapter 2, this includes a major shift in how we conduct exposures: rather than focusing on fear reduction during exposures (the old habituation model), we focus on the mismatch between what a child expects will occur (the feared consequence) and what actually occurs. This mismatch has been found to be critical for new learning, which is the purpose of exposure-based therapy. We also know that when someone does exposures across many situations and combines related triggers, he learns to be less afraid in a more lasting way.

The occasional return of anxious feelings in a situation that was previously conquered can be a good thing (Craske et al. 2015). For example, children may become anxious about being anxious. They may worry about the return of anxiety even after it has been well managed for a long time. In that case, occasional spikes of anxiety reinforce a child's ability to learn that he can be okay in spite of anxiety. This has a net benefit of reducing anxiety over the long run.

Just because your child is triggered from time to time or develops a new worry does not mean he has relapsed or is in danger of doing so. A spike in anxiety shouldn't be interpreted as a sign of relapse. How you and he manage and respond to spikes determines whether he will relapse. Many factors can lead to a recurrence of fears or the growth of new fears. You cannot always determine which factor is affecting him, and ultimately, the factor is less important than how you and he deal with any resurgence of anxiety. The following are the factors I most commonly see that relate to increased anxiety:

- increase in unstructured time (vacations, weekends, changes in schedule)
- temporary absence of trigger situations (summer vacation)
- maturation and changes in hormones, especially in pubescent and menstruating girls (I am hard pressed to think of female patients who do not have an increase in the frequency and severity of anxiety symptoms before and often during the menstrual cycle.)
- lifestyle changes that expose your child to new situations or situations that trigger fears
- the waxing and waning nature of anxiety

Your child's brain has a proclivity to overreact and get stuck on particular fears. This proclivity does not go away; it is part of her genetic makeup. Although successfully completing this program may completely eliminate anxiety about the situations your child worked on, it is more likely that this work will only decrease the frequency and severity of her spikes. You must continue to help your child manage her fears and not fall back on old behaviors. In a sense, you must help keep her mind fit, much as an athlete must stay fit to perform a sport. You must help her maintain the mental muscle she developed through hard work doing exposures and eliminating avoidance and safety behaviors and rituals.

Additionally, since your child does have this neurobiological proclivity, it is possible that other fears may develop throughout his life. Through this program, you and your child have learned principles and techniques that will enable you both to manage his fears—old or new—so they do not manage him. You must never forget these skills.

After your child has successfully completed this program, his anxieties may be well managed, but the work is not finished. The following important tips will help keep his fears at bay and his coping skills sharp.

Continue to Use the Tools

You have the tools; now it is up to you and your child to use them or lose them. If your child doesn't use them regularly, they will not be available when she needs them. While working through this book, you have identified the tools you and your child find most effective. She also must work to maintain the objectivity and attitude of acceptance gained by knowing how her brain works and by nicknaming when she is triggered.

Keep the Learning Fresh by Practicing Exposures

Your child may have conquered fears about situations that rarely occur in his life. For example, he may have overcome a needle-injection phobia and gone on to successfully receive a flu shot. He is unlikely to have a real-life opportunity to face this trigger situation with regularity, and after a year of no exposure to shots, he may experience a resurgence of anxiety. Even if the anxiety is not as high as before doing exposures, I recommend he practice to keep the learning fresh.

To practice, refer back to all the exposures your child conducted. One way to do this is to write down the experiments on index cards and create an exposure practice deck. Have your child pick a card once every a week or two and have him conduct the experiment again, following the same guidelines as before.

Similarly, if your child hasn't faced a trigger situation for some time and you know that such a situation is upcoming, get back in shape by reviewing tools and practicing exposures.

Watch for Signs of Relapse

Be on the lookout for signs that your child's fears are resurging. As part of your relapse prevention strategy, identify with your child which signs he might notice first if his fears begin to resurface. Ask directly. "John, if Worry Monster were to start bugging you again, what do you think you'd notice first?" Usually, he will say that he might notice a higher fear rating in previously mastered situations. He might also note an increased urge to avoid trigger situations. The use of safety behaviors or rituals is another warning sign.

Assessing these first signs is important for a number of reasons. First, assessment makes you and your child aware that he needs to continue using all available tools to stay on top of anxiety. Second, early detection enables troubleshooting before matters escalate. Better to be prepared with a strategy to manage a situation than to be surprised by it. Lastly, consistent oversight reinforces the message that he needs to confront rather than retreat from fears.

Consider Reducing Rewards

You have likely used rewards to boost your child's motivation to face fears. As she becomes less burdened by her fears, you can gradually reduce the rewards. You may need to continue giving some while she traverses the relapse-prevention stages, especially if you sense she still needs to work hard at managing fears. This is an individual decision parents need to make. If you give too many rewards, they may no longer seem like rewards. But if you feel your child lacks motivation to continue using tools or doing exposures, you will be wise to continue rewarding her efforts. I am rarely concerned about overdoing it with rewards when they are well deserved. Remember: rewards motivate!

Know When and How to Seek Professional Help

If your child's symptoms are severe, very distressing, or disrupt his ability to engage in age-appropriate activities, I suggest you consult with an experienced CBT therapist. Another factor to consider regarding whether to seek professional support is your child's level of motivation. A motivated child will be a more cooperative partner than one with little motivation. Even if you decide to seek professional guidance, the program described in this book can help you help your child more effectively while in treatment.

If you determine professional help will be useful to you and your child, or if you simply wish to have some support and guidance, here are some guidelines that can help you make good decisions about whom to engage. When trying to locate a mental health professional, make sure he or she practices CBT. It is not sufficient that a therapist "does a little CBT" as part of his or her practice. Do not assume therapists are experienced in CBT just because they represent themselves to be.

- An experienced therapist will explain that CBT focuses on people's thoughts and behaviors.
- The treatment should focus on the here and now, not on the past.
- The therapist should emphasize an exposure-based treatment.
- Treatment should include homework between sessions.
- Therapeutic goals should be established by the mental health professional.

To ensure the CBT therapist has sufficient experience assessing and treating anxiety disorders, ask about the following areas.

1. Specialization and focus

Q: How many patients in your practice do you treat for a diagnosed anxiety disorder?

A: The therapist should indicate that a significant percentage (at least 50 percent) of his or her practice comprises such children.

Q: What disorders do you have expertise in treating?

A: A qualified therapist should not hesitate to discuss openly the specific disorders he or she regularly treats.

2. Description of therapeutic approach and goals

Q: What specifically do you do in sessions with your patients? What specifically do you do with patients who have OCD (or panic attacks, social anxiety, phobias, separation anxiety)?

A: Responses should emphasize exposure treatments for all anxiety disorders. If they do not, find a different therapist. If the therapist gives a vague response, therapy will also be vague. CBT is not vague. It is very specific, goal directed, and straightforward. An experienced CBT therapist should be able to explain clearly what therapy will be like and how she or he will work with you to identify and meet therapy goals. This should give you a sense of how much work you would need to do to meet your goals, and therefore you can set reasonable expectations for the duration of the treatment.

3.   Time frame for therapy

Q: How many sessions do you typically need with a patient to facilitate significant symptom reduction, based on the symptoms described?

A: Answers will vary, depending on the onset of the symptoms and the presence of additional symptoms, such as depression, and other factors. But you should hear that patients are treated in a relatively time-limited framework. Therapy does not typically go on for years, but only months and sometimes even just several sessions.

4. Use of medication

Q: When do you consider medication as an option in treatment?

A: An experienced CBT therapist will recommend medication in a number of instances: if a CBT program has been fully implemented, but symptom reduction has not been significant or if the child cannot participate in exposures due to extreme distress; if the child is in such extreme distress that she cannot engage in typical activities (attend school, socialize); or if the child has little motivation and strong resistance to participate in CBT, which is often the result of a long history of avoidance.

Appendix M (http://www.newharbing er.com/39539) contains a Therapist Vetting Form, which you can print out and use to help you choose a therapist for your child. Most areas in the United States do not have sufficient numbers of trained CBT therapists to meet the needs of anxious children. Be patient and persistent in your efforts to find the right therapist. Contact major university hospitals and training centers as well as clinicians in private practice.

Whether or not you decide to consult a CBT therapist, this book provides you with the information you need to be an educated player in your child's management of anxiety. The tools acquired through this program will help you and your child live a healthier, less stressful life. Instead of watching in frustration as he experiences debilitating anxiety, you can actively contribute to his wellness. Congratulate yourself on your newfound skills and feel confident in your ability to move forward in helping your child.

SUMMARY: What Did You Learn from This Chapter?

- Tracking your child's progress in eliminating avoidance and safety behaviors and in doing exposures or ERPs is crucial for success.

- You must assess your own progress in reducing and eliminating accommodating behaviors.
- Daily observations and more formal weekly check-ins are ways to track progress.
- Establish specified days and times for regular check-ins.
- You and your child will benefit from seeing the hard numbers and concrete evidence of her hard work.
- Relapse means your child goes back to engaging in many or all of the avoidance and safety behaviors or rituals she used to do.
- Watch for signs of relapse and guard against it by encouraging her to continue to use the tools she has learned and practice exposures when necessary.
- Reduce rewards when she doesn't need the extra motivation.
- Consult an experienced CBT clinician if her symptoms are very severe, cause extreme distress, disrupt her ability to engage in normal age-appropriate activities, or disrupt family life.

- Know that what you have learned in this book allows you to be an educated player in her management of anxiety.

Acknowledgments

It indeed takes a village for a busy mother, wife, psychologist, friend, and athlete to complete a project such as this book. I want to acknowledge and thank many members of this village.

I want to thank the parents and children with whom I have worked over the past fifteen years for inspiring me to write this book. My dear high school best friend, Casey Mickle, guided me through the initial drafts. My colleague Dr. Michael Tompkins kindly supported initial drafts and encouraged me to persevere and make the manuscript more user friendly. Jude Berman stepped in and did just that, along with gently keeping me ahead of deadlines. I truly could not have done this without all these people.

My gratitude to Camille Hayes and the team at New Harbinger for believing in the project and supporting a first-time author so graciously, and for their careful suggestions and guidance.

My greatest appreciation goes to my husband, Michael Walker, my constant partner and companion, who consistently supports me in almost everything I do, including writing this book. And finally, to my children, Wheeler Walker and Liam Walker, who near deadlines had to put up with a stressed-out mother, as well as to Maxwell Walker, my middle son, who passed away before this book was completed.

References

Abramowitz, J.S. 2013. "The Practice of Exposure Therapy: Relevance of Cognitive-Behavioral Theory and Extinction Theory." *Behavior Therapy* 44 (4): 548–58.

Allen, J.L., and R.M. Rapee. 2004. "Anxiety Disorders." In *Cognitive Behaviour Therapy for Children and Families,* edited by P. Graham, 2nd ed., 300–19. Cambridge, UK: Cambridge University Press.

American Academy of Child and Adolescent Psychiatry. 2013. *Obsessive-Compulsive Disorder in Children and Adolescents.* Retrieved from http://www.aacap.org/AACAP/Families_and_Youth/Facts_for_Families/FFF-Guide/Obsessive-Compulsive-Disorder-In-Children-And-Adolescents-060.aspx.

Anxiety and Depression Association of America. 2016. *Children and Teens.* Retrieved from https://www.adaa.org/living-with-anxiety/children.

Beck, A.T. 1979. *Cognitive Therapy and the Emotional Disorders.* New York, NY: Penguin.

Beidel, D.C., and S.M. Turner. 1997. "At Risk for Anxiety: I. Psychopathology in the Offspring of Anxious Parents." *Journal of the American Academy of Child and Adolescent Psychiatry* 36 (7): 918–24.

Craske, M.G., A.M. Waters, R.L. Bergman, B. Naliboff, O.V. Lipp, H. Negoro, and E.M. Ornitz. 2008. "Is Aversive Learning a Marker of Risk for Anxiety Disorders in Children?" *Behaviour Research and Therapy* 46 (8): 954–67.

Craske, M.G., M. Treanor, C.C. Conway, T. Zbozinek, and B. Vervliet. 2015. "Maximizing Exposure Therapy: An Inhibitory Learning Approach." *Behaviour Research and Therapy* 58: 10–23. doi: 10.1016/j.brat.2014.04.006.

Forsyth, J.P., G.H. Eifert, and V. Barrios. 2006. "Fear Conditioning in an Emotion Regulation Context: A Fresh Perspective on the Origins of Anxiety Disorders." In M.G. Craske, D. Hermans, and D. Vansteenwegen (Eds.), *Fear and Learning: From Basic Processes to Clinical Implications,* 133–53. Washington, DC: American Psychological Association.

Garcia, A.M., J.J. Sapyta, P.S. Moore, J.B. Freeman, M.E. Franklin, J.S. March, and E.B. Foa. 2010. "Predictors and Moderators of Treatment Outcome in the Pediatric Obsessive Compulsive Treatment Study (POTS I)." *Journal of the American Academy of Child and Adolescent Psychiatry* 49 (10): 1024–33.

Ginsburg, G.S. 2009. "The Child Anxiety Prevention Study: Intervention Model and Primary Outcomes." *Journal of Consulting and Clinical Psychology* 77 (3): 580–87.

Goenjian, A.K., E.P. Noble, A.M. Steinberg, D.P. Walling, S.T. Stepanyan, S. Dandekar, and J.N. Bailey. 2014. "Association of COMT and TPH-2 GEnes with DSM-5 Based PTSD Symptoms."

Journal of Affective Disorders 172: 472–78.

Holzschneider, K., and C. Mulert. 2011. "Neuroimaging in Anxiety Disorders." *Dialogues in Clinical Neuroscience* 13 (4): 453–61.

Kashani, J.H., A.F. Vaidya, S.M. Soltys, A.C. Dandoy, L.M. Katz, and J.C. Reid. 1990. "Correlates of Anxiety in Psychiatrically Hospitalized Children and Their Parents." *American Journal of Psychiatry* 147 (3): 319–23.

Kessler, R.C., P. Berglund, O. Demler, R. Jin, K.R. Merikangas, and E.E. Walters. 2005. "Lifetime Prevalence and Age-of-Onset Distributions of DSM-IV Disorders in the National Comorbidity Survey Replication." *Archives of General Psychiatry* 62 (6): 593–602. doi:10.1001/archpsyc.62.6.593.

Lissek, S., S. Rabin, R.E. Heller, D. Lukenbaugh, M. Geraci, D.S. Pine, and C. Grillon. 2010. "Overgeneralization of Conditioned Fear As a Pathogenic

Marker of Panic Disorder." *American Journal of Psychiatry* 167 (1): 47–55.

March, J.S., and K. Mulle. 1998. *OCD in Children and Adolescents: A Cognitive-Behavioral Treatment Manual.* New York, NY: Guilford.

Mendlowicz, M.V., and M.B. Stein. 2000. "Quality of Life in Individuals with Anxiety Disorders." *The American Journal of Psychiatry* 157 (5): 669–82.

Merikangas, K.R., L.C. Dierker, and P. Szatmari. 1998. "Psychopathology among Offspring of Parents with Substance Abuse and/or Anxiety Disorders: A High-Risk Study." *Journal of Child Psychology and Psychiatry* 39 (5): 711–20.

Merlo, L.J., H.D. Lehmkuhl, G.R. Geffken, and E.A. Stroch. 2009. "Decreased Family Accommodation Associated with Improved Therapy Outcome in Pediatric Obsessive-Compulsive Disorder." *Journal of Consulting and Clinical Psychology* 77 (2): 355–60.

National Institutes of Health. 2016. "Understanding Anxiety Disorders: When Panic, Fear, and Worries Overwhelm." *NIH News in Health.* Retrieved from h ttps://newsinhealth.nih.gov/issue/mar2 016/feature1.

Olatunji, B.O., J.M. Cisler, and D.F. Tolin. 2007. "Quality of Life in the Anxiety Disorders: A Meta-Analytic Review." *Clinical Psychology Review* 27: 572–81.

Padesky, C.A. 1993. "Socratic Questioning: Changing Minds or Guiding Discovery?" Keynote Address to European Congress of Behavioral and Cognitive Therapies, London, September 24.

Rachman, S. 1980. "Emotional Processing." *Behaviour Research and Therapy* 18 (1): 51–60.

Thirlwall, K., P.J. Cooper, J. Karalus, M. Voysey, L. Willetts, and C. Creswell. 2013. "Treatment of Child Anxiety Disorders Via Guided Parent-Delivered Cognitive-Behavioural Therapy:

Randomized Controlled Trial." *British Journal of Psychiatry* 203 (6): 436–44. doi:10.1192/bjp.bp.113.126698.

Tompkins, M.A. 2013. *Anxiety and Avoidance: A Universal Treatment for Anxiety, Panic, and Fear.* Oakland, CA: New Harbinger.

Trouche, S., J.M. Sasaki, T. Tu, and L.G. Reijmers. 2013. "Fear Extinction Causes Target-Specific Remodeling of Perisomatic Inhibitory Synapses." *Neuron* 80 (4): 1054–65. doi:10.1016/j.neuron.2013.07.047.

Wagner, A.P. 2005. *Worried No More: Help and Hope for Anxious Children.* 2nd ed. Apex, NC: Lighthouse Press.

Zbozinek, T.D., E.A. Holmes, and M.G. Craske. 2015. "The Effect of Positive Mood Induction on Reducing Reinstatement Fear: Relevance for Long Term Outcomes of Exposure Therapy." *Behaviour Research and Therapy* 71: 65–75.

Bridget Flynn Walker, PhD, is a graduate of the University of California, Berkeley. Walker received her PhD from the California School of Professional Psychology in 1991. In addition to fellowships at UCLA, Norwalk Hospital, and Kaiser Permanente, Walker completed a two-year postdoctoral fellowship with Jeffrey Martin, PhD—an anxiety disorder specialist and professor at UCSF School of Medicine. For the past fifteen years, Walker's private practice has focused exclusively on assessing and treating children, adolescents, and adults with anxiety disorders, and on training other mental health professionals to do the same using cognitive behavioral therapy (CBT). Walker's consultation and teaching services are requested by mental health professionals throughout the San Francisco Bay Area, and she is frequently asked to educate and guide school professionals in San Francisco and Marin counties. Walker works closely with a team of pediatricians at Golden Gate Pediatrics, and regularly consults with leaders of the San

Francisco Psychotherapy Research Group.

Foreword writer **Michael A. Tompkins, PhD, ABPP,** is founding partner of the San Francisco Bay Area Center for Cognitive Therapy, Diplomate of the Academy of Cognitive Therapy, and assistant clinical professor at the University of California, Berkeley. He is author of five books, including *OCD* and *Digging Out.*

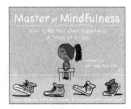
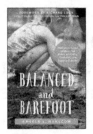
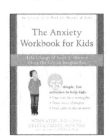

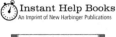
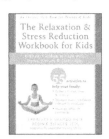
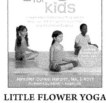
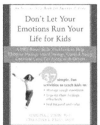

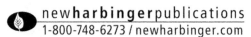

Back Cover Material

Practical, Proven Solutions to Take Charge of Your Child's Anxiety

If your child has anxiety, you know how difficult it can be to navigate daily situations at home, in school, or with friends. It hurts to see your child afraid or constantly worried and missing out on the best parts of life. So, how can you manage your child's anxiety during those challenging moments and restore peace and balance to both your lives?

Written by a psychologist and expert in childhood anxiety, Anxiety **Relief for Kids provides** quick, in-the-moment solutions you can easily use at home, in social settings, or anywhere anxiety takes hold. You'll find an overview of the different types of anxiety disorders, learn how to identify your child's coping behaviors, and uncover the triggers that set your child of. Most importantly, you'll discover tailored, scientifically proven interventions for your child's specific symptoms. If you're struggling with how to help your anxious child, the practical strategies in this book will help you find the solutions you need.

"Just what the doctor ordered! ... This book provides a real-life tool kit that will help families and their physicians ease the fears that children often have."—LAUREL J. SCHULTZ, MD, MPH, community pediatrician at Golden Gate Pediatrics in San Francisco, CA

Bridget Flynn Walker, PhD, has a private practice that focuses on assessing and treating children, adolescents, and adults with anxiety disorders. In addition, her consultation and teaching services are requested by mental health professionals in and around San Francisco, CA, where she resides.

Foreword writer **Michael A. Tompkins, PhD, ABPP**, is a licensed psychologist who practices in Oakland, CA.

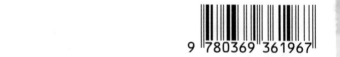

9 780369 361967